- Clinical Nutr.
  1995   3-15

- Nutr. Reviews
  96   31-33

Nutritional Management
of Genetic Disorders

CURRENT CONCEPTS IN NUTRITION

Myron Winick, Editor

Institute of Human Nutrition
Columbia University College of Physicians and Surgeons

NUTRITIONAL MANAGEMENT OF GENETIC DISORDERS

Edited by

MYRON WINICK

Institute of Human Nutrition
Columbia University College of Physicians and Surgeons

A WILEY-INTERSCIENCE PUBLICATION
JOHN WILEY & SONS
New York • Chichester • Brisbane • Toronto

Library of Congress Cataloging in Publication Data:

Main entry under title:
Nutritional management of genetic disorders.,

  (Current concepts in nutrition; v. 8)
  "A Wiley-Interscience publication."
  Includes bibliographical references and index.
  1. Metabolism, Inborn errors of—Diet therapy.
2. Metabolism, Inborn errors of—Nutritional aspects.
3. Medical genetics. I. Winick, Myron. II. Series.

RC627.8.N87   616.3′9′042   79-16192
ISBN 0-471-05781-9

Printed in the United States of America

10 9 8 7 6 5 4 3 2 1

Preface

A great number of recent discoveries in the field of genetic diseases, especially those involving inborn errors of metabolism, have had important nutritional consequences, especially as related to the treatment of patients. In many of these diseases the abnormality consists of a genetic defect in the body's ability to metabolize a particular nutrient. The result, depending on exactly where the defect occurs, may range from a full blown deficiency of the nutrient in question, for example, vitamin D-resistant rickets, to a specific syndrome arising from an abnormality in a single pathway normally traversed by that nutrient, for example, vitamin B_{12}-dependent methylmalonic aciduria.

Other serious diseases have a genetic component in their etiology but cannot be classified as "pure" genetic diseases. The successful treatment of some of these diseases, such as diabetes mellitus, lactose intolerance, cystic fibrosis, and some of the hyperlipidemias, requires very specific nutritional management.

Finally, there are certain diseases which are primarily environmental but which are much more serious in genetically susceptible hosts. Atherosclerotic heart disease is one such disease in which the environmental factors are multiple; obesity is another in which the single most important factor is nutritional.

This volume is an attempt to bring together the most current knowledge in this complicated field. Even as I write this preface, our knowledge is being increased, and no doubt some of our concepts will change. Hence this represents a description of the current "state of the art" in an exciting and relatively new area.

The opening chapter is a discussion of vitamin D-resistant rickets. Its author, Dr. Hector DeLuca, has contributed much of the information currently available which demonstrates that the active vitamin, 1,25-dihydroxyvitamin D_3, is synthesized in the kidney from a precursor, 25-hydroxyvitamin D_3, which had been previously synthesized in the liver from vitamin D_3 in the diet or supplied by the skin after exposure to ultraviolet light. Hence this vitamin undergoes two major transformations before it becomes physiologically active. The actual rate of synthesis of the active form in the kidney is controlled by a complex mechanism involving body calcium metabolism. Thus 1,25-dihydroxyvitamin D_3 is actually a hormone synthesized by the kidney which acts primarily on the gastrointestinal tract, controlling calcium absorption. Genetic inability to synthesize this hormone exists, producing a picture similar to vitamin D deficiency rickets. However the disease does not respond to normal doses of vitamin D (since the active form cannot be synthesized from this precursor). In the past, this disease was treated with huge doses of vitamin D_3, which could partly overcome the block either by contributing small amounts of activity itself or by stimulating some synthesis of 1,25-dihydroxyvitamin D_3. Such therapy was at best palliative and carried with it the risks of vitamin D toxicity. Now, however, specific therapy has become available since 1,25-hydroxyvitamin D_3 can be supplied. Thus, vitamin D-resistant rickets is a genetic disease, involving the metabolism of an essential nutrient (vitamin D_3), which is converted in two steps to an active hormone (1,25-dihydroxyvitamin D_3), which in turn is involved in the absorption of another essential nutrient, calcium.

Inborn errors involving the metabolism of other nutrients are not as clearly worked out as with vitamin D and usually specific replacement therapy is not available. The next three chapters are devoted to inborn errors of amino acid metabolism and discuss three different approaches to the management of these diseases depending on the exact nature of the defect. The first approach is best demonstrated in phenylketonuria, a disease in which the enzyme necessary for the conversion of phenylalanine to tyrosine is not active. Therefore, too much phenylalanine builds up in the body. This substance is toxic, especially to the brain, and tyrosine is deficient. Clinically, the major problem is the high levels of phenylalanine. Since all proteins are mixtures of amino acids, there is no natural way to keep the quantity of phenylalanine in the diet extremely low. Hence synthetic low phenylalanine diets are used. This requires careful management, since the patient is walking a fine line between protein deficiency and its attendant growth failure and phenylalanine toxicity and its accompanying mental retardation. There are other metabolic errors of amino acid metabolism much rarer than phenylketonuria and somewhat more complicated, such as maple syrup urine disease, which are treated by using the same therapeutic approach.

The second group of amino acid disorders are those involving errors in amino acid metabolism because of inability to utilize certain cofactors properly. This may be due to an inability to synthesize a particular apoenzyme or to improper absorption or metabolic conversion of the vitamin cofactor itself. For example, all of the pyridoxine (B_6)-responsive inborn errors are due to faulty apoenzyme production. The B_{12}-responsive metabolic errors are due both to faulty apoenzyme production and to abnormalities in the utilization of vitamin B_{12} itself. All of these abnormalities are "leaky"; that is, they can be "overpowered" with high doses of the vitamin cofactor. Thus these abnormalities, if diagnosed early, can be successfully treated using high doses of the appropriate vitamin.

The third group of amino acid disturbances are those involving abnormalities in the urea cycle. To date all of these have been due to the absence of activity of one or another enzyme in the cycle. Precursors prior to the block accumulate, and the most significant of these is ammonia. Products after the block are decreased and may have to be supplied in the diet. A new form of therapy has been tried recently and seems to be useful. It involves the use of α keto analogs of certain amino acids. The theory is that ammonia will be taken up by these analogs by transamination, forming the appropriate amino acids, which can then be used in protein synthesis. In addition, this therapy will reduce the nitrogen load presented to the kidney and hence reduce the "need" for the urea cycle. Although the long term experience with this form of therapy is extremely limited, results at present suggest that in fact these changes do occur. Hence the outlook for the future of this form of therapy is optimistic.

The next section of the book deals with genetic abnormalities of carbohydrate metabolism. Two chapters discuss specific abnormalities causing lactose intolerance or intolerance to other carbohydrates. Three chapters are concerned with the most common and in some cases the most complicated of the carbohydrate group with genetic overtones, diabetes mellitus.

Lactose intolerance is more of a physiologic state than a disease, since a majority of the people of the world suffer from it. In these individuals, the activity of the enzyme lactase declines with age, and ingestion of lactose produces symptoms of flatulence, pain, and diarrhea. The major question, however, is whether the amount of lactose in one or two glasses of milk is sufficient to produce symptoms in older children, especially black children, who in the United States undergo this change at an earlier age than most white children. The implications of this question from the standpoint of such programs as school lunches and breakfasts are obvious.

Intolerance of other carbohydrates, though much rarer than lactose intolerance, can occur. These can involve lower levels of the other disaccharidases; in some cases they occur for unknown reasons. Such patients will often exhibit ileitis-like symptoms, which respond to the removal of the offending sugar.

Diabetes mellitus is a disease that is partly genetic in origin. To fully understand the genetics of this disease we must first separate diabetes into its two major types, maturity onset and juvenile onset. The maturity-onset diabetes is by far the more common and appears to be inherited as an autosomal dominant. The time of appearance and the severity, however, will vary. The juvenile type appears to be recessive, not for the disease but for susceptibility to the disease. Moreover, there is a direct correlation between juvenile diabetes and a genetically determined antigen system located on the surface of human lymphocytes (HLA). These data plus epidemiologic data suggest that juvenile diabetes is a viral disease that manifests itself in a genetically susceptible population marked by a particular genotype which is expressed in the HLA system. This entire concept is new but represents certainly one of the most intriguing areas in diabetes research.

In treating the diabetic, whether adult or juvenile onset, diet is extremely important. In the typical adult-onset diabetic, total calories should be controlled, since in obese patients weight reduction alone may control the diabetes. The timing of meals is also extremely important, especially in juvenile diabetics being treated with insulin. Five feedings per day are recommended, and in this case caloric intake should be adequate. In both types of diabetes, cholesterol and saturated fat should be reduced. This translates into a substitution of carbohydrate for fat, and hence a proper diabetic diet will be relatively high in carbohydrate.

The management of the pregnant diabetic presents a special case. The tendency toward ketosis during pregnancy and the need for adequate weight gain by the mother for adequate fetal growth limits the amount of caloric restriction that can be employed. Carbohydrate intake should be relatively constant from day to day and should be in a relatively unrefined form that maximizes the intake of associated fiber. However, the mainstay of therapy in the pregnant diabetic is insulin.

The last section of this volume deals with lipids, first in terms of obesity and second in terms of the hyperlipidemias. There is no clear picture at present of the role genetics plays in human obesity. In animals, there are genetic types of obesity. Both hyperplastic and hypertrophic obesity occur on a genetic basis. In humans, while studies certainly show that obesity runs in families, it is difficult to demonstrate a strictly genetic effect. The data at present would suggest that most obesity, regardless of whether it is predominantly hyperplastic or hypertrophic, is environmentally induced. However, there is certainly the possibility that a small proportion of obese individuals manifest the abnormality as a result of a "genetic" defect or at least have a "genetic tendency" to be obese. The identification of this particular group could be extremely important, since the therapeutic approach might be quite different from that for environmentally induced obesity.

The diseases with high levels of serum lipids which have a genetic component are the last group to be discussed. A new and very exciting technique has been developed in which cultured fibroblasts are used and their ability in vitro to synthesize cholesterol is monitored. By using this technique metabolic defects in cholesterol metabolism can be pinpointed. Genetic defects can be characterized by using this tissue culture method. For example, in patients with the homozygous form of receptor-negative familial hypercholesterolemia the fibroblasts lack functional low density lipoprotein (LDL) receptors. The cells, therefore, fail to bind LDL properly. Unable to utilize LDL cholesterol, these cells satisfy their cholesterol requirement by synthesizing large amounts of cholesterol de novo, even when high levels of LDL are present in the culture medium.

The ability to analyze the genetic defect carefully in various familial types of hyperlipidemias should open new approaches to both diagnosis and management.

The diet for patients with hyperlipidemia is the same whether the cause is genetic, dietary, or both—low saturated fat, low cholesterol intake. In any patient with hyperlipidemia a restriction of dietary cholesterol to amounts under 300g/day is recommended.

The final chapter discusses a serious genetic disease, cystic fibrosis. These patients, because of fat malabsorption, will have low serum lipid levels, may develop essential fatty acid (EFA) deficiency, and may be depleted of fat-soluble vitamins. One such vitamin is vitamin E. In a group of patients with chemical evidence of EFA deficiency in their serum, supplementation with corn oil and vitamin E was undertaken. The blood chemistries returned rapidly to normal but what was more striking was that the sweat electrolytes, which are abnormal in this disease, as manifested by high sweat sodium chloride, returned toward the normal range. These data need confirmation but could represent an important step toward a better understanding of the pathophysiology of cystic fibrosis. Moreover, obvious therapeutic avenues are suggested by these findings.

In summary, this book explores in depth some of the relationships between genetic diseases and diet. It emphasizes those genetic diseases whose management depends on the use of important nutritional principles in management. It is certainly not complete, nor is it intended to be. However the physician or nutritionist confronted by certain genetic diseases should get an understanding of basic nutritional principles used in their management.

MYRON WINICK

New York, New York
September 1979

Contents

Nutritional Management
of Genetic Disorders

PART 1

Vitamins

1

Vitamin D-Resistant Rickets
A Prototype of Nutritional
Management of a Genetic Disorder

HECTOR F. DELUCA, PH.D.

Department of Biochemistry, College of Agricultural and Life Sciences, University of
Wisconsin-Madison, Madison, Wisconsin

During the decade beginning in 1920 came the discovery of vitamin D
(1,2) and, in particular, the production of vitamin D by ultraviolet
irradiation of foods and plant sterols (3,4), which led to the elimination
of a major medical problem; namely, rickets among children in the
northern hemispheres. Although this vitamin D seemed to protect the
major segment of the population, it did not totally eliminate rachitic
conditions, which continued to appear despite vitamin D supplementation. Thus mention of vitamin D-resistant rickets began to appear in the
clinical literature and it is now recognized that there are as many as 33
different types of vitamin D-resistant rickets among children (5).
Indeed, many of these are rare and it is beyond our scope to discuss
them here. Interested readers are directed elsewhere for a survey of
these different conditions (5).

During the past decade has come the major discovery that vitamin D
must be metabolically converted to an active form before it can carry out
its functions (6). Pursuit of this problem has led to the identification of
an endocrine system based in the kidney which produces a hormone that
in turn regulates calcium and phosphorus metabolism (6–8). In true
hormonal fashion, the biogenesis of this hormone is strongly feedback
regulated by the need for calcium and the need for phosphorus (6,7). It

This work supported by a grant from the National Institutes of Health, No. AM-14881,
and the Harry Steenbock Research Fund.

3

has become increasingly apparent, therefore, that a number of bone pathologies could result from a defect in the vitamin D endocrine system (9). This chapter will illustrate some of the more clearly defined conditions and will discuss the use of the vitamin D metabolites in the nutritional management of patients suffering from these conditions.

Vitamin D must be regarded as a prohormone which is normally produced in skin by ultraviolet irradiation of 7-dehydrocholesterol (Fig. 1). Because insufficient amounts of ultraviolet light reach the skins of many people, it is important that vitamin D be provided by dietary means. This chapter will demonstrate that vitamin D is converted to an active steroid-type hormone, which carries out its functions in the classical steroid hormone sense; namely, by a receptor mechanism that provides for the transcription of mRNA. This mRNA is believed to code for calcium and phosphorus transport proteins. We must therefore regard the entire vitamin D system as a steroid endocrine system rather than merely regarding vitamin D as a classical vitamin supplement.

VITAMIN D METABOLISM

Through the application of modern tools of chemistry and biochemistry has come the realization that vitamin D must be metabolically converted to an active form before it can carry out its functions (6,7). During the past decade and a half, the pathway shown in Figure 1 has been elucidated in great detail (10). Each of the intermediates in the metabolic conversions has been isolated in pure form, chemically identified, and chemically synthesized (6,7,10). There exists in the epidermis an abundant supply of 7-dehydrocholesterol, which undergoes a chemical photolysis reaction to yield presumably previtamin D, which undergoes a thermally dependent isomerization to vitamin D_3. Vitamin D_3 has been isolated in pure form from the skins of animals irradiated with ultraviolet light, and the antirachitic substance produced in the skin therefore is clearly vitamin D_3 (11,12). It is of some importance that the reaction in skin does not appear to require a protein or an enzyme and that it is very much a chemical photolysis reaction not unlike that which occurs in organic solvents. Nevertheless, this reaction should be kept in mind by physicians who wish to treat patients suffering from fat malabsorption syndromes in that this method can be used to provide vitamin D more conveniently than the troublesome parenteral method.

Vitamin D_3, whether taken in the diet or made in the skin, rapidly accumulates in the liver. This accumulation is unique among the D vitamins, since it does not occur for any of the metabolites subsequent to

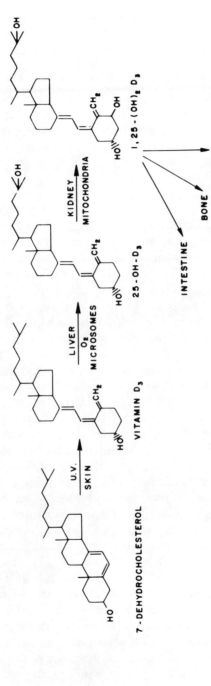

Figure 1. Metabolic alterations required for vitamin D activity.

5

vitamin D_3. In the liver, vitamin D_3 is hydroxylated on carbon-25 to form 25-hydroxyvitamin D_3 (25-OH-D_3) (13,14). This reaction occurs in the endoplasmic reticulum and requires NaDPH and molecular oxygen (15), but its enzymatic characteristics have not been fully explained. Although it is feedback regulated by the hepatic level of 25-OH-D_3 (16), this regulation is of limited capacity, since administration of large amounts of vitamin D_3 will produce increasing amounts of 25-OH-D_3 in the plasma. The 25-OH-D_3 is the major circulating form of vitamin D in the plasma, present at about 30 ng/ml. Vitamin D_3 itself circulates at levels much lower than that, on the order of 1 to 2 ng/ml. All vitamin D compounds circulate bound to an α_2-globulin of about 52,000 M.W. which has been isolated in pure form from rats (17) and man (18,19). The binding protein is present in huge excess over the circulating metabolites (20), which suggests that it must have still some other function besides transporting the vitamin D molecules.

The 25-OH-D_3 is taken up by the kidney, where it undergoes an additional and obligatory reaction to form 1,25-dihydroxyvitamin D_3 (21–23). This reaction occurs in the mitochondria in chickens and requires NaDPH, molecular oxygen, and magnesium ions (24,25). This reaction is indeed a cytochrome P-450-dependent reaction and its three components have been isolated and recombined to provide a reconstituted system (26,27). The enzymatic machinery of this reaction is very similar to the steroidogenesis system in the adrenal glands. The reaction which occurs in the kidney is found in that organ exclusively, which forms the basis for the idea that 1,25-$(OH)_2D_3$ is a true hormone. The 1,25-$(OH)_2D_3$ which is formed in the kidney is then transported to the target tissues, where it initiates calcium and phosphorus transport reactions. Table 1 illustrates the basic finding which demonstrates that 1,25-$(OH)_2D_3$ is the metabolically active form of the vitamin and that since it is formed exclusively in the kidney and has its function in target organs of intestine and bone it must be regarded a hormone. Table 1 demonstrates that nephrectomy but not uremia caused by uretary ligation six hours prior to the experiment will prevent the conversion of 25-OH-D_3 to the 1,25-$(OH)_2D_3$, a discovery originally made by Kodicek (21) and quickly confirmed in our laboratory (23). Since nephrectomy prevents the conversion of 25-OH-D_3 to the 1,25-$(OH)_2D_3$, this tool could be used to examine the question of whether the target organs of intestine and bone will respond directly to 25-OH-D_3 when given at physiologic doses. The results for the intestinal tests are illustrated in Table 1. It is clear that in animals which have a high degree of uremia but which retain their renal tissue, the response of the intestine to 25-OH-D_3 can be observed. On the other hand, nephrectomy prevents the

Table 1   The Necessity for Kidney Tissue for Expression of 25-OH-D_3 but Not 1,25-$(OH)_2D_3$ Activity

	1,25-$(OH)_2D_3$ Synthesis	Stimulation of Calcium Absorption by	
		25-OH-D_3	1,25-$(OH)_2D_3$
No renal tissue	$--$	$--$	$+++$
Acutely impaired renal function	$+++$	$++$	$+++$

response of intestine to the 25-OH-D_3 (28,29). The 1,25-$(OH)_2D_3$ produces a response whether kidneys are present or not. Similar experiments have been carried out with the intestinal phosphate transport reaction (30,31) and with the mobilization of calcium from bone (32). These results demonstrate clearly that 1,25-$(OH)_2D_3$ or a further metabolite must be the physiologically active form of vitamin D rather than 25-OH-D_3 or vitamin D_3 itself. It is not possible to exclude completely the possibility that 1,25-$(OH)_2D_3$ is further converted in the target tissues to tissue active forms, but so far that has not been demonstrated.

Besides the conversion of vitamin D to 1,25-$(OH)_2D_3$ as described above, there are other important metabolic reactions of the vitamin D molecule. The most significant and the most studied is that of 24R-hydroxylation of 25-OH-D_3 and the 1,25-$(OH)_2D_3$ as shown in Figure 2. It is known that in the kidney (33) and in the intestine (34) there exists a potent 25-OH-D_3 and 1,25-$(OH)_2D_3$-24R-hydroxylase. This enzyme is absent in the vitamin D-deficient animal and is induced by the active hormone, 1,25-$(OH)_2D_3$ (35). The exact role of 24-hydroxylation is not known, although it is evident that 24-hydroxylation does not increase biological activity in any of the systems known to be responsive to vitamin D (36–38). In fact, in most cases there is a diminished biological activity, which strongly supports the idea that 24-hydroxylation may be the initial event in the inactivation of the potent vitamin D molecule. Much is known about the 24-hydroxylation reaction and there is much speculation about a possible functional role of the 24-hydroxylated vitamins. Interested readers are directed elsewhere (39), but so far none of the studies that purport to demonstrate special activity of the 24-hydroxylated vitamins have adequate foundations. For

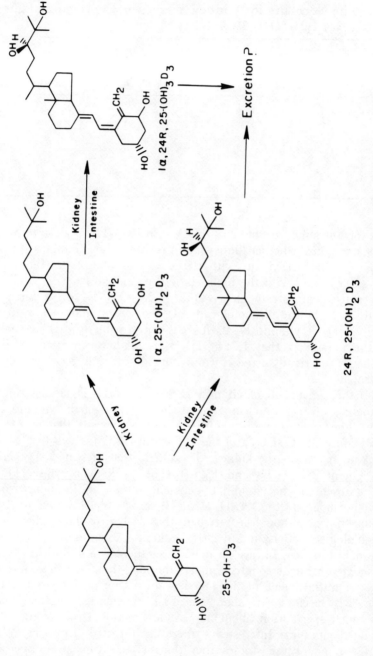

Figure 2. The 24R-hydroxylation of either 25-OH-D₃ or 1,25-(OH)₂D₃ to give the corresponding 24R-hydroxylated forms of vitamin D, which are believed to be the initial intermediates in the inactivation of the active forms of vitamin D.

our purpose here we can regard the 24-hydroxylation as an inactivation reaction.

FUNCTIONS OF 1,25-(OH)$_2$D$_3$

The known metabolic functions of 1,25-(OH)$_2$D$_3$ are illustrated in Figure 3. It is known that 1,25-(OH)$_2$D$_3$ is responsible for the elevation of intestinal calcium absorption, long known as a function of vitamin D. This is an active calcium transport process in which calcium is transported against an electrochemical potential gradient and which involves phosphate as the accompanying anion, although this is not mandatory (40–42). In addition to this mechanism, 1,25-(OH)$_2$D$_3$ also initiates an independent phosphate transport mechanism which is especially evident in the distal segments of the small intestine (30,43–45). This phosphate-oriented system is also an active transport system and requires sodium (46). However, sodium is apparently required on the initial uptake phase rather than on the extrusion phase. In addition to the functions in the small intestine, 1,25-(OH)$_2$D$_3$ is required together with the parathyroid hormone to permit the mobilization of calcium from the bone fluid compartment to the extracellular fluid compartment (47). This mechanism is the prime one for protection against hypocalcemic tetany. In addition, parathyroid hormone and 1,25-(OH)$_2$D$_3$ improve renal reabsorption of calcium (48,49). In the absence of these two hormones 99% of the filtered calcium is reabsorbed anyway and thus the remaining 1% is that which is acted upon by 1,25-(OH)$_2$D$_3$ and the parathyroid hormone. Although this may appear to be a small effect quantitatively, it must be borne in mind that adult humans filter as

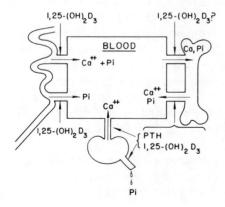

Figure 3. Sites of action of 1,25-(OH)$_2$D$_3$ and the parathyroid hormone in the regulation of calcium and phosphorus metabolism.

much as 7 to 10 g of calcium per day so 1% of this figure is not an insignificant amount. Of some interest is the idea that $1,25\text{-}(OH)_2D_3$ and the parathyroid hormone both cause a phosphate diuresis (50). In the case of $1,25\text{-}(OH)_2D_3$, the phosphate diuresis is found only under conditions of hyperphosphatemia.

The elevations of plasma calcium and plasma phosphorus are responsible for the correction of hypocalcemic tetany on one hand and the rachitic bone lesions on the other (9). There are some unexplained clinical studies which suggest that $1,25\text{-}(OH)_2D_3$ may have a direct effect on the mineralization process, but so far direct biochemical or physiological evidence for this remains to be produced.

REGULATION OF $1,25\text{-}(OH)_2D_3$ BY CALCIUM

In 1971 Boyle et al. (51) demonstrated that animals on a low calcium diet accumulated large amounts of $1,25\text{-}(OH)_2D_3$ in their intestines and plasma whereas those on a high calcium diet accumulated primarily 24,25-dihydroxyvitamin D_3 $(24,25\text{-}(OH)_2D_3)$. Further examination of this question revealed that there was an important relationship between serum calcium concentration and the accumulation of $1,25\text{-}(OH)_2D_3$ in the plasma (52). Animals which had slight hypocalcemia accumulated large amounts of $1,25\text{-}(OH)_2D_3$ and no $24,25\text{-}(OH)_2D_3$ whereas those which were hypercalcemic accumulated no $1,25\text{-}(OH)_2D_3$ and instead accumulated the $24,25\text{-}(OH)_2D_3$. Omdahl et al. (53) demonstrated that this regulation was a direct regulation of the 1-hydroxylase and the 24-hydroxylase as measured in vitro. Thus the need for calcium stimulated the 25-hydroxyvitamin D_3-1α-hydroxylase in the kidney and suppressed 24-hydroxylase in kidney and presumably in intestine. Since it is known that hypocalcemia is sensed by the parathyroid glands, which in response to hypocalcemia secrete parathyroid hormone, it seemed reasonable to suspect that the parathyroid hormone might be the mediator of the hypocalcemic signal to the 25-OH-D_3-1-hydroxylase (54). Examination of this point demonstrated clearly that the hypocalcemic stimulation of $1,25\text{-}(OH)_2D_3$ production was indeed mediated by the parathyroid glands and parathyroid hormone secretion. Thus parathyroidectomy of hypocalcemic animals resulted in a diminished 25-OH-D_3-1-hydroxylase, which could be restored by the exogenous injection of $1,25\text{-}(OH)_2D_3$ (54,55).

Since $1,25\text{-}(OH)_2D_3$ is a major calcium-mobilizing hormone, both from bone and from intestine, it became of interest to learn whether the effects of parathyroid hormone are entirely mediated by increased biogenesis of $1,25$-$(OH)_2D_3$ (47). Thus it has been shown that the improved intestinal calcium absorption which results from parathyroid hormone administration is the direct result of increased production of $1,25$-$(OH)_2D_3$, and parathyroid hormone itself does not participate directly in the intestine to stimulate intestinal calcium absorption. On the other hand, the mobilization of calcium from bone requires both the parathyroid hormone and the $1,25$-$(OH)_2D_3$.

With these discoveries it became possible to re-examine the calcium homeostatic mechanism and include the vitamin D endocrine system in this regulatory system (56). This system is summarized in Figure 4. Thus hypocalcemia brings about increased parathyroid hormone secretion. The parathyroid hormone is then found to bind specifically to kidney and bone (57,58). In the kidney it causes a phosphate diuresis and in the presence of endogenous $1,25$-$(OH)_2D_3$ it improves renal reabsorption of calcium. In addition, it stimulates the 25-OH-D_3-1α-hydroxylase, which produces increased amounts of $1,25$-$(OH)_2D_3$. This hormone then proceeds to the intestine where, by itself, it stimulates intestinal calcium absorption. In the bone, it, together with the parathyroid hormone, stimulates the mobilization of calcium from bone. These three sources of calcium then bring about an elevation of plasma calcium concentration, resulting in a shutdown of parathyroid hormone secretion, which in turn shuts down the entire calcium-mobilizing system.

It is known that calcium in the plasma must be very quickly regulated and, in addition, there must be a mechanism whereby one can regulate the utilization of dietary or environmental calcium. The $1,25$-$(OH)_2D_3$ system is a very slow reacting system, requiring hours following initial stimulation before $1,25$-$(OH)_2D_3$ appears in the circulation (54) and, in addition, hours are required for $1,25$-$(OH)_2D_3$ to stimulate intestine and bone (59). On the other hand, parathyroid hormone is secreted within minutes following stimulation and its action as well as its lifetime can be measured in minutes (60). Thus in an acute need for calcium, the parathyroid hormone which is secreted will act on the kidney to stimulate renal reabsorption of calcium in the presence of an endogenous $1,25$-$(OH)_2D_3$. Similarly, at the bone site, it will mobilize calcium from bone with the existent $1,25$-$(OH)_2D_3$. This will bring about a correction of plasma calcium concentration without the reaction of 1-hydroxylase. However, it is obvious that this response ultimately relies on the skeletal calcium. If there is a protracted perturbation or need for calcium, then the resulting chronically elevated parathyroid hormone secretion stimulates $1,25$-$(OH)_2D_3$ production. The $1,25$-$(OH)_2D_3$ then sensitizes the kidney and the bone to parathyroid hormone secretion; but in addition,

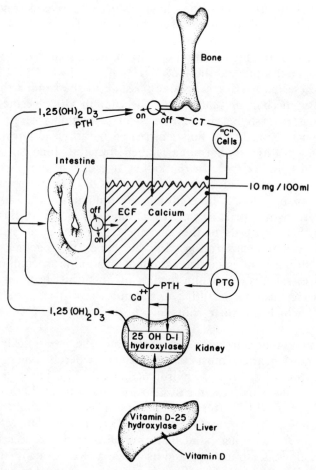

Figure 4. The calcium homeostatic mechanism represented diagrammatically. When the extracellular fluid calcium level falls below normal, it triggers the parathyroid glands to secrete parathyroid hormone. This hormone then stimulates the kidney to reabsorb calcium and stimulates the renal 25-OH-D₃1-hydroxylase. The resulting 1,25-$(OH)_2D_3$ proceeds to the intestine, where it stimulates intestinal calcium absorption, and to the bone where, together with parathyroid hormone, it stimulates the mobilization of calcium from the bone fluid compartment. Not shown on the figure is the idea that 1,25-$(OH)_2D_3$ also functions with the parathyroid hormone in stimulating renal reabsorption of calcium. These three sources of calcium cause extracellular fluid calcium to rise to the normal range, which then shuts off parathyroid hormone secretion.

12

it causes the intestine to increase its efficiency of absorption. Thus the ability of the intestine to adapt to dietary calcium needs is regulated by parathyroid hormone and 1,25-$(OH)_2D_3$, as shown in Figure 5. This regulation has been totally confirmed by the fact that exogenous parathyroid hormone (61) or exogenous 1,25-$(OH)_2D_3$ (62) or both completely eliminate the ability of the intestine to adapt to dietary calcium. Hence the famous Nicolaysen's endogenous factor (63), which was known to instruct the intestine of the needs of the skeleton for calcium, is the parathyroid hormone–1,25-$(OH)_2D_3$ system.

REGULATION OF VITAMIN D METABOLISM BY DIETARY AND PLASMA PHOSPHORUS CONCENTRATION

As was demonstrated earlier, 1,25-$(OH)_2D_3$ plays an important role in stimulating intestinal phosphate absorption and in the mobilization of phosphate from bone (64). This brings about an increased plasma phosphorus concentration which is necessary for mineralization of bone (65) and muscle function. Therefore an important function of 1,25-$(OH)_2D_3$

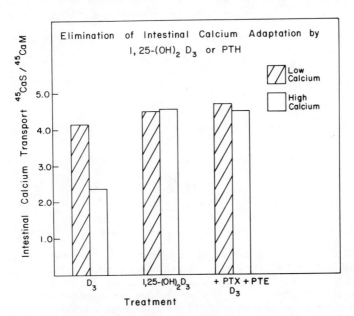

Figure 5. The elimination of the ability of the intestinal calcium absorption system to adapt to dietary calcium levels by the administration of 1,25-$(OH)_2D_3$ or parathyroid hormone from exogenous sources.

is to improve the transport of phosphate both in intestine and in bone. It is therefore reasonable to suspect that plasma phosphate may have a marked influence on the metabolism of vitamin D. It was demonstrated by Tanaka et al. (66) that the accumulation of $1,25\text{-}(OH)_2D_3$ is markedly increased under conditions of phosphate depletion. It was possible, therefore, to demonstrate clearly the regulation of $1,25\text{-}(OH)_2D_3$ accumulation in the plasma by plasma phosphate concentration. To do this it was necessary to remove the calcium-regulating system by thyroparathyroidectomy. One could then adjust plasma phosphate concentration by dietary deprivation or by glucose loading as shown in Figure 6 (66). Under conditions of normal plasma phosphorus, which in the young growing rat is 9 mg/dl, no $1,25\text{-}(OH)_2D_3$ is made. Instead, $24,25\text{-}(OH)_2D_3$ is made. If these thyroparathyroidectomized animals are then made hypophosphatemic by the means suggested above, they begin to accumulate $1,25\text{-}(OH)_2D_3$ in their plasma and intestines. Thus the need for phosphorus stimulates the accumulation of this phosphate-mobilizing hormone. The mechanism whereby $1,25\text{-}(OH)_2D_3$ accumulates in phosphate depletion is not entirely clear (67–69). There is a stimulation of the $25\text{-}OH\text{-}D_3\text{-}1\alpha$-hydroxylase (70) but there must be some additional effect on $1,25\text{-}(OH)_2D_3$ metabolism to permit this accumulation. In addition, phosphate depletion also sensitizes the intestine

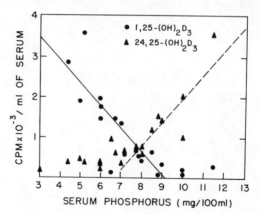

Figure 6. The relationship between serum inorganic phosphorus levels and accumulation of either $24,25\text{-}(OH)_2D_3$ or $1,25\text{-}(OH)_2D_3$ from $25\text{-}OH\text{-}D_3$ in thyroparathyroidectomized rats. Rats are thyroparathyroidectomized and placed on diets of varying phosphorus levels. After they adapt to this regimen they are injected with radioactive $25\text{-}OH\text{-}D_3$ and the amount of radioactive $24,25\text{-}(OH)_2D_3$ or radioactive $1,25\text{-}(OH)_2D_3$ that accumulates in the plasma during a 6- or 12-hour period is plotted versus serum phosphorus concentration. These results demonstrate that even in the absence of parathyroid glands, hypophosphatemia will stimulate accumulation of $1,25\text{-}(OH)_2D_3$ in the serum.

to 1,25-(OH)$_2$D$_3$ (62). Hence it is important to recognize that phosphate depletion can play an important role in regulating 1,25-(OH)$_2$D$_3$ metabolism. Furthermore, 1,25-(OH)$_2$D$_3$ must be recognized as a phosphate-mobilizing hormone.

REGULATION OF VITAMIN D METABOLISM BY OTHER ENDOCRINE SYSTEMS

It is known that there are some extraordinary demands for calcium under certain physiologic circumstances. Thus under conditions of rapid growth, or under conditions of lactation, or in the case of birds during egg production, when there is a great demand for calcium for eggshells, it is apparent that there must be some mechanism permitting the mobilization of calcium for these purposes. There is increasing evidence that the mechanism which underlies the utilization of these extraordinary amounts of calcium is the vitamin D endocrine system. As an example, it is instructive to illustrate the mechanism whereby calcium is mobilized for eggshell production in birds. It is known that there is a marked elevation of the 25-OH-D$_3$-1-hydroxylase in birds laying eggs as compared to their male counterparts or their resting female counterparts (71,72). In examining this question more closely it became apparent that the sex hormones may well influence the 25-OH-D$_3$-1-hydroxylase. Thus injection of estradiol into mature male birds brings about a suppression of the 24-hydroxylase and a marked elevation of the 1-hydroxylase, which is followed by an increase in plasma calcium concentration (Fig. 6). This elevation requires the presence not only of estradiol but also of testosterone or progesterone (72–74). All three hormones act synergistically to bring about a marked elevation of the 25-OH-D$_3$-1-hydroxylase. It seems clear that the resulting increased 1,25-(OH)$_2$D$_3$ plays an important role in the mobilization of medullary bone and in increased intestinal calcium absorption which attends egg production and eggshell formation (74). The details of this mechanism are now being worked out to explain the interplay of the hormones that brings about these amazing shifts in calcium metabolism. Other evidence has been presented which suggests that growth hormone and prolactin may also stimulate the 25-OH-D$_3$-1-hydroxylase and account for the increased utilization of calcium necessary under these circumstances (75). Therefore, it may be that other endocrine systems which bring about metabolic shifts requiring calcium may impinge upon the vitamin D endocrine system to permit this calcium mobilization. It is also apparent that diseases may result from defective regulatory systems involving the hormones which bring about the increased $1,25\text{-}(OH)_2D_3$ production.

RACHITOGENESIS

With the background of the sites of action of $1,25\text{-}(OH)_2D_3$ and the regulation of its production, one can begin to examine rachitogenesis in the light of what has been historically observed. Of particular importance is a study by Fraser et al. (76) in 1967, which demonstrated three phases of rachitogenesis (Figure 7). In stage one, there is a hypocalcemia with no apparent metabolic bone disease. Plasma phosphate is approximately normal. In this first stage of rachitogenesis vitamin D begins to be depleted, which begins to retard intestinal calcium absorption, but there is still enough vitamin D to support mobilization of calcium from bone. In the second phase of rachitogenesis the parathyroid glands have reacted to the hypocalcemia brought about by inadequate calcium absorption, producing a secondary hyperparathyroidism. This results in a phosphate diuresis which is parathyroid hormone dependent. This in turn results in a fall in plasma phosphate

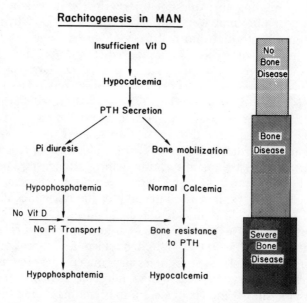

Figure 7. The sequence of events giving rise to bone disease during vitamin D depletion in children.

concentration, but because the parathyroid hormone in increasing amounts can mobilize calcium from bone, the hypocalcemia is corrected. The second phase shows normal plasma calcium and low plasma phosphorus concentration. It is at this stage that bone disease begins to appear as a result of the hypophosphatemia (76). In the third stage of rachitogenesis, the patient is depleted of vitamin D so that no longer is bone mobilized in response to the excessive secretions of parathyroid hormone. Thus the patient becomes hypocalcemic. However, the large amount of parathyroid hormone which circulates causes a phosphate diuresis, giving low plasma phosphorus concentration. This is aggravated by low phosphorus absorption brought about by the lack of 1,25-$(OH)_2D_3$, and florid rickets is then obtained. These investigators believe that the primary reason for the pathological rickets is low plasma phosphorus concentration. In fact, evidence has been provided that infusion of phosphate will heal the rickets, although it is unclear whether it will heal it completely. In rats, rachitogenesis can be reproduced only with a double deficiency of phosphate and of vitamin D (71,77). Therefore, one can consider that rickets is largely a phosphate deficiency disease. With this background, we can begin to discuss the genetically determined vitamin D-resistant rachitic conditions.

VITAMIN D-DEPENDENCY RICKETS: A TRUE METABOLIC BLOCK IN VITAMIN D METABOLISM

This disease, which was discovered by Prader et al. (78), is autosomal recessive and the children present with amino aciduria, and with rickets exactly similar to the rickets of vitamin D deficiency despite normal intakes of vitamin D. Furthermore, this disease can be completely corrected by the administration of large amounts of vitamin D of the order of 50,000 to 100,000 units/day. With the discovery of the pathway of vitamin D metabolism necessary for function, it was of some interest to determine whether one of these enzymatic conversions might be defective (79). Administration of 25-OH-D_3 provided for healing of the rickets, but pharmacological amounts of this form of vitamin D were required. Furthermore, circulating levels of 25-OH-D_3 are normal in these patients. Of considerable importance was the demonstration that this disease could be cured by the administration of physiologic amounts of 1,25-$(OH)_2D_3$ (Figure 8). Furthermore, recent analyses of the plasma levels of 1,25-$(OH)_2D_3$ clearly show this disease to have an attendant low circulating level of this hormone. It therefore appears, as shown in Figure 9, that this disease represents a true defect in the conversion of

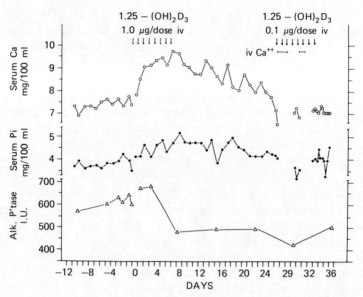

Figure 8. The response of a vitamin D depencency rickets patient to intravenous 1,25-(OH)₂D₃. It is important to note that even after 7 days of intravenous 1,25-(OH)₂D₃ at 1 μg/day, clear mineralization of bone could be observed radiologically.

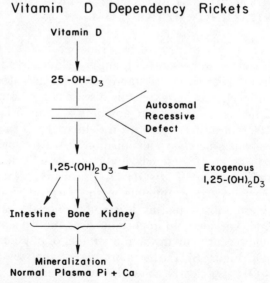

Figure 9. Metabolic block in vitamin D-dependency rickets and its correction by exogenous 1,25-(OH)₂D₃.

25-OH-D_3 to the 1,25-$(OH)_2D_3$. It can be cured by physiologic amounts of 1,25-$(OH)_2D_3$, but of considerable interest is the fact that it can be cured with either vitamin D_3 or 25-OH-D_3. Figure 10 illustrates an important bit of information which shows that these patients in fact have low levels of circulating 1,25-$(OH)_2D_3$ and when they are healed by the administration of 25-OH-D_3 in pharmacological amounts, the plasma levels of 1,25-$(OH)_2D_3$ do not rise. It has recently been demonstrated that the receptor mechanism of the small intestine will react to large amounts of 25-OH-D_3 (80,81). Thus 25-OH-D_3 can act as an analog of 1,25-$(OH)_2D_3$ in the target tissue. Therefore, by giving large amounts of 25-OH-D_3 one can bypass the requirement for conversion to the 1,25-$(OH)_2D_3$. In any case, this disease, which is quite rare, can be very conveniently managed with the active form of vitamin D given as a nutritional supplement under carefully controlled conditions. It should be recognized that 1,25-$(OH)_2D_3$ is not subject to the controls of vitamin D_3 and hence this compound must be used very carefully on patients so as to prevent unwanted hypercalcemia.

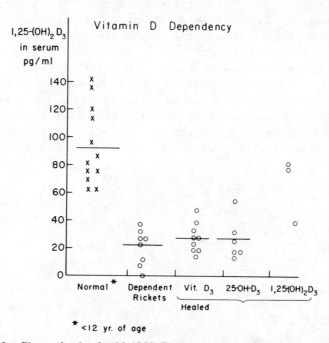

Figure 10.   Plasma levels of 1,25-$(OH)_2D_3$ in normal children and in children with vitamin D-dependency rickets. Note that healing the patients with vitamin D or 25-OH-D_3 does not elevate plasma 1,25-$(OH)_2D_3$ levels. Not shown here is the fact that plasma 25-OH-D_3 levels in these treated children become very high.

X-LINKED DOMINANT VITAMIN D-RESISTANT HYPOPHOSPHATEMIC RICKETS: A DEFECT IN PHOSPHATE METABOLISM

This is the most common of the genetically determined vitamin D-resistant rachitic conditions known (82). The genetics are well worked out and the patients present with hypophosphatemia, rickets, normal plasma calcium levels, normal to low circulating parathyroid hormone levels (83), amino aciduria, and of considerable interest, in most clinical conditions, low rates of intestinal calcium absorption. Work by Scriver and others (84–86) has demonstrated that the primary defect in this disease is a phosphate transport defect in the renal tubular cells (Fig. 11) in which there is a lack of phosphate reabsorption. More recently, using the animal model (87), it has been shown that there is a defect in phosphate absorption in the small intestine (88) in agreement with the work in man (85). It is likely that there is a generalized defect in phosphate transport reactions, resulting in low plasma phosphate concentration. It is curious that this disease is accompanied by low rates of calcium absorption, when one would predict high levels of intestinal calcium absorption (82). More recent work by Scriver (personal communication) has suggested that the defect in phosphate transport is at the basal-lateral membrane of the renal tubular cell (Fig. 12) in which there is a defect in the exit of phosphate from the absorption cells. It is therefore possible that the accumulation of phosphate in these cells may suppress production of $1,25\text{-}(OH)_2D_3$ and, in fact, work with Rasmussen and our group has shown that in many cases of this disease there is a low circulating level of $1,25\text{-}(OH)_2D_3$. Therefore, although

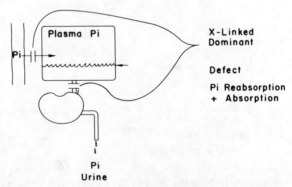

Figure 11.   The defect in phosphate transport reactions in patients suffering from X-linked dominant familial hypophosphatemic vitamin D-resistant rickets (VDRR).

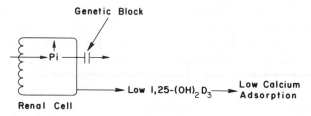

Figure 12. Proposed secondary defect in calcium metabolism in patients suffering from the X-linked hypophosphatemic vitamin D-resistant rickets.

this disease is not a defect in vitamin D metabolism, there is certainly an impairment of the vitamin D metabolic regulation system. Treatment, as shown in Figure 13, is best accomplished by replacement of the phosphate by large oral doses of phosphate given very frequently during the day (89,90). Clinicians tell me that about 1 to 1.5 g/day of oral phosphate given at frequent intervals is very helpful in treatment of this disease. Furthermore, the poor calcium absorption and the tendency to secondary hyperparathyroidism brought about by phosphate supplementation can be corrected by the administration of $1,25\text{-}(OH)_2D_3$ at about 1 μg/day. It is important, however, that this be very carefully titrated so that the optimal level of $1,25\text{-}(OH)_2D_3$ is achieved. Using this approach, several groups are reporting not only improved mineralization of bone and correction of the rachitic condition, but an improvement in the growth response (90,91). Lack of growth is, of course, an important feature of this disease.

VITAMIN D RESISTANCE OF RENAL FAILURE

A discussion of management of vitamin D-resistant rickets would be incomplete without saying something about rickets secondary to chronic

```
            Treatment:  VDRR

1.  Oral Phosphate - 1.-1.5 g/day in
    frequent doses compensate for
    loss of phosphate.

2.  1,25-(OH)2D3 to correct calcium
    defect.

3.  Care to adjust correct dose of
    1,25-(OH)2D3.
```

Figure 13. Treatment protocol for patients suffering from the hypophosphatemic vitamin D-resistant rickets.

43730

renal failure. Although this is not a genetic defect in vitamin D metabolism, certainly in many circumstances, renal failure is the result of a genetic defect. Figure 14 illustrates some of the problems one encounters during the course of renal failure. The major problem is, of course, the loss of nephrons. This brings about a loss of the major phosphate-excreting organ, resulting in phosphate retention (92). In addition, the loss of nephrons brings about a lack of $1,25\text{-}(OH)_2D_3$, which is further aggravated by phosphate retention. This results in a low rate of calcium absorption, contributing to hypocalcemia. Hypocalcemia then triggers parathyroid gland hyperplasia and gives secondary hyperparathyroidism, which will result in destruction of bone as long as $1,25\text{-}(OH)_2D_3$ is present even in small amounts. In addition, failure of calcium absorption and mineralization causes rickets and poor growth. Figure 15 illustrates the steps taken in treatment of chronic renal failure with the use of the vitamin D metabolites. It is essential that the phosphate of the plasma be adjusted to normal levels. This is done by phosphate deprivation and, if necessary, aluminum-magnesium hydroxide gel (phosphate binders) may be provided. It is important to keep the phosphate level normal and not below normal. If the phosphate level is below normal, mineralization of newly forming bone will fail (93). On

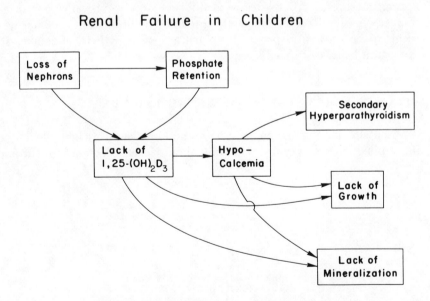

Figure 14.   The pathogenesis of renal osteodystrophy.

TREATMENT - RENAL FAILURE

1. Phosphate restriction + phosphate
   binders ──→ normal serum Pi.

2. Adequate calcium intake.

3. If PTG are autonomous--partial
   PTX.

4. 1,25-(OH)$_2$D$_3$ (or analog) at
   0.05 µg/kg.

Figure 15.   Treatment of children having rickets secondary to chronic renal failure.

the other hand, if it is above normal, soft tissue calcification, secondary hyperparathyroidism, and suppression of 1,25-(OH)$_2$D$_3$ production in the remaining nephrons will exist. Next, one must be sure that the parathyroid glands have not become autonomous and that the glands are responsive to increased plasma calcium concentration. If they are autonomous and do not respond, it is possible that partial parathyroidectomy will be required before treatment can begin. Following these adjustments, treatment with 1,25-(OH)$_2$D$_3$ is initiated. Figure 16a illustrates rickets in a patient who had a combination of Fanconi syndrome and chronic renal failure and Figure 16b illustrates the response of the patient to 1,25-(OH)$_2$D$_3$ therapy (Chesney and DeLuca, submitted). There is no question that these patients respond very well (94) and that this type of management results in phenomenal improvement in growth as shown by the Tanner Growth Velocity Curve.

HYPOPARATHYROIDISM—A DEFECT IN THE SIGNAL FOR VITAMIN D METABOLISM

Obviously, hypoparathyroidism is a condition in which the patient cannot sense hypocalcemia. As a result, parathyroid hormone is absent and consequently, production of 1,25-(OH)$_2$D$_3$ in response to the need for calcium does not take place (94,95). This results in a skeleton that cannot yield its calcium to correct hypocalcemia and an intestine that has no 1,25-(OH)$_2$D$_3$ to improve its intestinal calcium absorption. These patients are best treated by the administration of 1 g/day of oral calcium plus about 1 µg/day of 1,25-(OH)$_2$D$_3$ (95,97). Figure 17 illustrates the response of such a patient to 1 µg/day of 1,25-(OH)$_2$D$_3$. This patient was resistant to even 750,000 units of vitamin D daily and, as can be seen, was nicely managed with 1,25-(OH)$_2$D$_3$ at 1 µg/day.

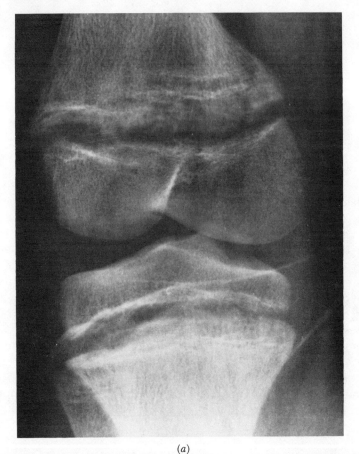

(a)

Figure 16a. X-ray of the knee of a child with Fanconi syndrome and chronic renal failure. Note the severe rachitic lesions.

The patient became hypercalcemic with 2 μg/day and has been kept well managed on the 1-hydroxylated vitamins for long periods of time without difficulty. There are some hypoparathyroid patients who do not respond well to low doses of 1,25-$(OH)_2D_3$ but can be managed with doses of up to 5 μg/day of 1,25-$(OH)_2D_3$. It is important to note that dietary calcium is required for 1,25-$(OH)_2D_3$ to correct the hypocalcemia of hypoparathyroidism because the bone fluid calcium is not available even to a patient given 1,25-$(OH)_2D_3$ because of the lack of parathyroid hormone and because both parathyroid hormone and 1,25-$(OH)_2D_3$ are required for this mobilization response.

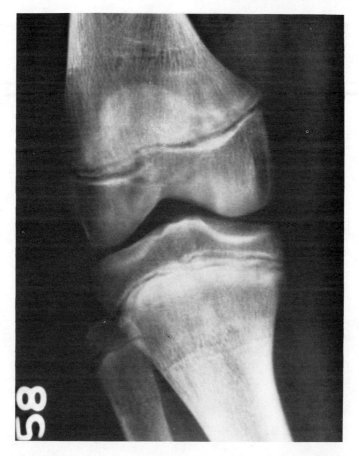

Figure 16b.   The same child after 24 months of 1 µg/day of 1α-25-(OH)₂D₃. There is no question that the skeletal lesions have been normalized in the child suffering from this condition. Not shown is the fact that this child showed remarkable catch-up growth response.

HYPOCALCEMIA OF THE PREMATURE INFANT

Hypocalcemia is a significant problem in premature infants. This is probably the result of premature parathyroid glands and premature kidneys, which are unable to make 1,25-(OH)₂D₃, as shown in Figure 18. These children also show considerable difficulty in mineralizing their skeletons. In studies with Fraser (98) and Tsang (in preparation)

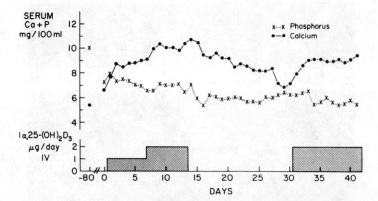

Figure 17. The response of a hypoparathyroid (idiopathic) child to 1α-25-(OH)$_2$D$_3$. This patient had been on 750,000 units/day of vitamin D$_2$ with chronic hypocalcemia. The patient responded to 1μg/day of 1,25-(OH)$_2$D$_3$ as shown in the figure (see Kooh et al. (96)).

we have been able to demonstrate an impressive correction of the hypocalcemia of these premature infants with 1,25-(OH)$_2$D$_3$. Data from Tsang's group is shown in Figure 19, demonstrating that children respond very well to 1,25-(OH)$_2$D$_3$.

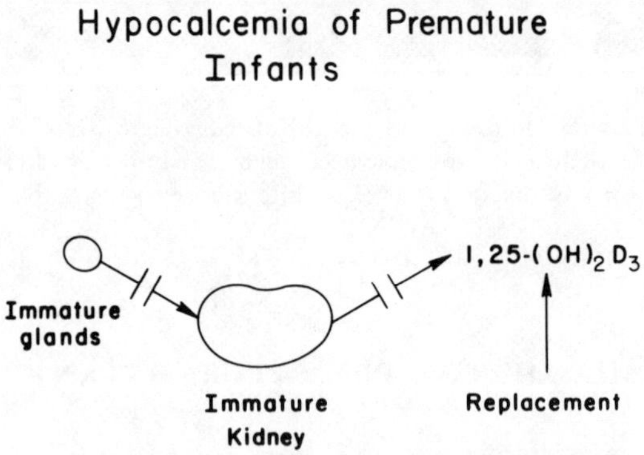

Hypocalcemia of Premature Infants

Figure 18. The possible causes of immature parathyroid glands or immature kidneys or both, giving rise to insufficient amounts of 1,25-(OH)$_2$D$_3$. This results in hypocalcemic tetany and often a prolonged delay in bone mineralization and formation. Treatment with 1,25-(OH)$_2$D$_3$ at 1μg/child/day has been effective in correcting these disturbances.

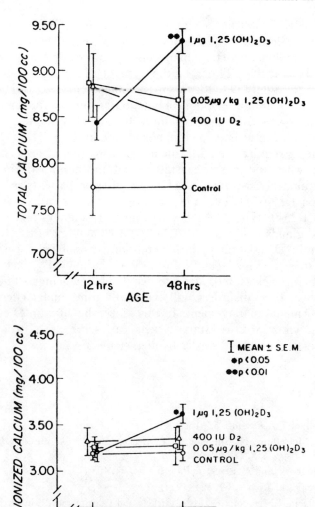

Figure 19. The response of hypocalcemic premature infants to 1 μg/day of 1,25-(OH)$_2$D$_3$. These data were collected by Dr. R. Tsang of the University of Cincinnati.

SUMMARY AND CONCLUSIONS

The discovery of the vitamin D endocrine system has opened up many possibilities in our understanding of metabolic bone disease. Of particular importance is the fact that we can now manage certain genetic disorders resulting in vitamin D-resistant rickets or vitamin D-resistant hypocalcemia with the new active hormonal forms of vitamin D and with intelligent dietary management to provide for correction of the mineral difficulty. Thus, in the case of vitamin D dependency, replacement need only be with the missing hormone, $1,25\text{-}(OH)_2D_3$. On the other hand, familial hypophosphatemia requires adjustment of the plasma phosphorus by frequent administration of oral phosphate and the adjustment of intestinal calcium absorption by $1,25\text{-}(OH)_2D_3$. Renal failure patients require the adjustment of plasma phosphorus concentration and parathyroid hormone status, and the administration of the missing hormone $1,25\text{-}(OH)_2D_3$. Hypoparathyroid patients require oral calcium plus $1,25\text{-}(OH)_2D_3$, and premature infants require administration of the $1,25\text{-}(OH)_2D_3$ because the immature kidneys and immature parathyroid glands fail to produce the required amount of this hormone. Other vitamin D-resistant rachitic conditions cannot be discussed here for lack of space and for lack of information. Undoubtedly, such patients as those having rickets secondary to renal tubular acidosis and rickets secondary to hepatic disorders will eventually come under effective dietary and hormonal management. In this sense, the vitamin D endocrine system and vitamin D-resistant rickets can serve as a prototype of management of a genetic disorder by dietary means.

REFERENCES

1. E. Mellanby, *J. Physiol.*, **52**, 1iii (1919).
2. E. V. McCollum, N. Simonds, J. E. Becker, and P. G. Shipley, *Bull. Johns Hopkins Hosp.*, **33**, 229 (1922).
3. H. Steenbock, and A. Black, *J. Biol. Chem.*, **61**, 405 (1924).
4. H. Steenbock, *Science,* **60**, 224 (1924).
5. C. E. Dent, "Metabolic Forms of Rickets and Osteomalacia," in H. Bickel and J. Stern, Eds., *Inborn Errors of Calcium and Bone Metabolism,* MTP Press Ltd., Lancaster, 1977, p. 124.
6. H. F. DeLuca, *Fed. Prod.*, **33**, 2211 (1974).
7. J. L. Omdahl and H. F. DeLuca, *Physiol. Rev.*, **53**, 327 (1973).
8. E. Kodicek, *Lancet,* **1**, 325 (1974).
9. H. F. DeLuca, *Ann. Royal College of Physicians and Surgeons of Canada,* pp. 216–25 (1977).
10. H. F. DeLuca and H. K. Schnoes. *Ann. Rev. Biochem.*, **45**, 631 (1976).
11. R. P. Esvelt, H. F. DeLuca, and H. K. Schnoes, "The Production of Vitamin D_3 in Ultraviolet Irradiated Rat Skin," in *Proc. 6th Parathyroid Conference,* (abs.) Excerpta Medica, Amsterdam (in press).

12. M. F. Holick, J. E. Frommer, S. C. McNeill, N. M. Richtand, J. W. Henley, and J. T. Potts, Jr., *Biochem. Biophys. Res. Commun.*, **76**, 107 (1977).

13. G. Ponchon, A. L. Kennan, and H. F. DeLuca, *J. Clin. Invest.*, **48**, 2032 (1969).

14. M. Horsting and H. F. DeLuca, *Biochem. Biophys. Res. Commun.*, **36**, 251 (1969).

15. M. Bhattacharyya and H. F. DeLuca, *Arch. Biochem. Biophys.*, **160**, 58 (1974).

16. M. Bhattacharyya and H. F. DeLuca, *J. Biol. Chem.*, **248**, 2969 (1973).

17. K. M. Botham, J. G. Ghazarian, B. E. Kream, and H. F. DeLuca, *Biochemistry*, **15**, 2130 (1976).

18. J. G. Haddad and J. Walgate, *J. Biol. Chem.*, **251**, 4803 (1976).

19. M. Imawari, K. Kida, and D. S. Goodman, *J. Clin. Invest.*, **58**, 514 (1976).

20. J. G. Haddad, L. Hillman, and S. Rojanasathit, *J. Clin. Endocrinol. Metab.*, **43**, 86 (1976).

21. D. R. Fraser and E. Kodicek, *Nature*, **228**, 764 (1970).

22. M. F. Holick, H. K. Schnoes, H. F. DeLuca, T. Suda, and R. J. Cousins, *Biochemistry*, **10**, 2799 (1971).

23. R. Gray, I. Boyle, and H. F. DeLuca, *Science*, **172**, 1232 (1971).

24. R. W. Gray, J. L. Omdahl, J. G. Ghazarian, and H. F. DeLuca, *J. Biol. Chem.*, **247**, 7528 (1972).

25. J. G. Ghazarian and H. F. DeLuca, *Arch. Biochem. Biophys.*, **160**, 63 (1974).

26. J. G. Ghazarian, C. R. Jefcoate, J. C. Knutson, W. H. Orme-Johnson, and H. F. DeLuca, *J. Biol. Chem.*, **249**, 3026 (1974).

27. J. I. Pedersen, J. G. Ghazarian, N. R. Orme-Johnson, and H. F. DeLuca, *J. Biol. Chem.*, **251**, 3933 (1976).

28. I. T. Boyle, L. Miravet, R. W. Gray, M. F. Holick, and H. F. DeLuca, *Endocrinology*, **90**, 605 (1972).

29. R. G. Wong, A. W. Norman, C. R. Reddy, and J. W. Coburn, *J. Clin. Invest.*, **51**, 1287 (1972).

30. T. C. Chen, L. Castillo, M. Korycka-Dahl, and H. F. DeLuca, *J. Nutr.*, **104**, 1056 (1974).

31. M. W. Walling, "1,25-Dihydroxyvitamin D_3 and Intestinal Phosphate Absorption," in A. W. Norman, K. Schaefer, J. W. Coburn, H. F. DeLuca, D. Fraser, H. G. Grigoleit and D. v. Herrath, Eds., *Vitamin D: Biochemical, Chemical and Clinical Aspects Related to Calcium Metabolism*, Walter de Gruyter, Berlin, 1977, p. 321.

32. M. F. Holick, M. Garabedian, and H. F. DeLuca, *Science*, **176**, 1146 (1972).

33. J. C. Knutson and H. F. DeLuca, *Biochemistry*, **13**, 1543 (1974).

34. H. F. DeLuca and H. F. Schnoes, "Recent Advances in Our Understanding of the Metabolism and Mechanism of Action of 1,25-Dihydroxyvitamin D_3," in *Proc. 6th Parathyroid Conference*, Excerpta Medica, Amsterdam (in press).

35. Y. Tanaka, R. S. Lorenc, and H. F. DeLuca, *Arch. Biochem. Biophys.*, **171**, 521 (1975).

36. M. F. Holick, L. A. Baxter, P. K. Schraufrogel, T. E. Tavela, and H. F. DeLuca, *J. Biol. Chem.*, **251**, 397 (1976).

37. M. F. Holick, A. Kleiner-Bossaler, H. K. Schnoes, P. M. Kasten, I. T. Boyle, and H. F. DeLuca, *J. Biol. Chem.,* **248,** 6691 (1973).

38. Y. Tanaka, H. F. DeLuca, N. Ikekawa, M. Morisaki, and N. Koizumi, *Arch. Biochem. Biophys.,* **170,** 620 (1975).

39. *Vitamin D: Biochemical, Chemical and Clinical Aspects Related to Calcium Metabolism,* A. W. Norman, K. Schaefer, J. W. Coburn, H. F. DeLuca, D. Fraser, H. G. Grigoleit, and D. v. Herrath, Eds., Walter de Gruyter, Berlin, 1977.

40. D. L. Martin and H. F. DeLuca, *Arch. Biochem. Biophys.,* **134,** 139 (1969).

41. T. H. Adams and A. W. Norman, *J. Biol. Chem.,* **245,** 4421 (1970).

42. M. W. Walling and S. S. Rothman, *Am. J. Physiol.,* **217,** 1144 (1969).

43. H. E. Harrison and H. C. Harrison, *Am. J. Physiol.,* **201,** 1007 (1961).

44. S. Kowarski and D. Schachter, *J. Biol. Chem.,* **244,** 211 (1969).

45. R. H. Wasserman and A. N. Taylor, *J. Nutr.,* **103,** 586 (1973).

46. A. N. Taylor, *J. Nutr.,* **104,** 489 (1974).

47. M. Garabedian, Y. Tanaka, M. F. Holick, and H. F. DeLuca, *Endocrinology,* **94,** 1022 (1974).

48. R. A. L. Sutton, C. A. Harris, N. L. M. Wong, and J. Dirks, "Effects of Vitamin D on Renal Tubular Calcium Transport," in A. W. Norman, K. Schaefer, J. W. Coburn, H. F. DeLuca, D. Fraser, H. G. Grigoleit and D. v. Herrath, Eds., *Vitamin D: Biochemical, Chemical and Clinical Aspects Related to Calcium Metabolism,* Walter De Gruyter, Berlin, 1977, p. 451.

49. C. R. Kleeman, D. Bernstein, R. Rockney, J. T. Dowling, and M. H. Maxwell, "Studies on the Renal Clearance of Diffusible Calcium and the Role of the Parathyroid Glands in its Regulation," in R. O. Greep and R. V. Talmage, Eds., *The Parathyroids,* Thomas, Springfield, 1961, p. 353.

50. J.-P., Bonjour and H. Fleisch, "The Effects of Vitamin D and Its Metabolites on the Renal Handling of Phosphate," in A. W. Norman, K. Schaefer, J. W. Coburn, H. F. DeLuca, D. Fraser, H. G. Grigoleit, and D. v. Herrath, Eds., *Vitamin D: Biochemical, Chemical and Clinical Aspects Related To Calcium Metabolism,* Walter de Gruyter, Berlin, 1977, p. 419.

51. I. T. Boyle, R. W. Gray, and H. F. DeLuca, *Proc. Nat. Acad. Sci. USA,* **68,** 2131 (1971).

52. I. T. Boyle, R. W. Gray, J. L. Omdahl, and H. F. DeLuca, "Calcium Control of the *in vivo* Biosynthesis of 1,25-Dihydroxyvitamin D_3: Nicolaysen's Endogenous Factor," in S. Taylor, Ed., *Endocrinology 1971,* Heinemann, London, 1972, p. 468.

53. J. L. Omdahl, R. W. Gray, I. T. Boyle, J. Knutson, and H. F. DeLuca, *Nature New Biol.,* **237,** 63 (1972).

54. M. Garabedian, M. F. Holick, H. F. DeLuca, and I. T. Boyle, *Proc. Nat. Acad. Sci. USA,* **69,** 1673 (1972).

55. D. R. Fraser and E. Kodicek, *Nature New Biol.,* **241,** 163 (1973).

56. H. F. DeLuca, *Acta Orthop. Scand.,* **46,** 286 (1975).

57. J. E. Zull and D. W. Repke, *J. Biol. Chem.,* **247,** 2195 (1972).

58. M. W. Neuman, W. F. Neuman, and K. Lane, *Calcif. Tiss. Res.,* **18,** 289 (1975).

59. Y. Tanaka and H. F. DeLuca, *Arch. Biochem. Biophys.*, **146**, 574 (1971).

60. *Calcium Regulating Hormones*, R. V. Talmage, M. Owen, and J. A. Parsons, Eds., Excerpta Medica, American Elsevier, New York, 1975.

61. M. L. Ribovich and H. F. DeLuca, *Arch. Biochem. Biophys.*, **175**, 256 (1976).

62. M. L. Ribovich and H. F. DeLuca, *Arch. Biochem. Biophys.*, **170**, 529 (1975).

63. R. Nicolaysen, N. Eeg-Larsen, and O. J. Malm, *Physiol. Rev.*, **33**, 424 (1953).

64. L. Castillo, Y. Tanaka, and H. F. DeLuca, *Endocrinology*, **97**, 995 (1975).

65. Y. Tanaka and H. F. DeLuca, *Proc. Nat. Acad. Sci. USA*, **71**, 1040 (1974).

66. Y. Tanaka and H. F. DeLuca, *Arch. Biochem. Biophys.*, **154**, 566 (1973).

67. H. F. DeLuca, "Regulation of Vitamin D Metabolism in the Kidney," in S. G. Massry and E. Ritz, Eds., *Phosphate Metabolism,* Plenum, New York, Vol. 81, 1977, p. 195.

68. A. W. Norman, E. J. Friedland, and H. Henry, "Interrelationships Between the Key Elements of the Vitamin D Endocrine System: 25-OH-D_3-1-Hydroxylase, Serum Calcium and Phosphorus Levels, Intestinal 1,25-$(OH)_2D_3$, and Intestinal Calcium Binding Protein," in S. G. Massry and E. Ritz, Eds., *Phosphate Metabolism,* Vol. 81, Plenum, New York, 1977, p. 211.

69. M. Haussler, M. Hughes, D. Baylink, E. T. Littledike, D. Cork, and M. Pitt, "Influence of Phosphate Depletion on the Biosynthesis and Circulating Level of 1α,25-Dihydroxyvitamin D," in S. G. Massry and E. Ritz, Eds., *Phosphate Metabolism,* Vol. 81, Plenum, New York, 1977, p. 233.

70. L. A. Baxer and H. F. DeLuca, *J. Biol. Chem.*, **251**, 3158 (1976).

71. Y. Tanaka, L. Castillo and H. F. DeLuca, *Proc. Nat. Acad. Sci. USA*, **73**, 2701 (1976).

72. L. Castillo, Y. Tanaka, H. F. DeLuca, and M. L. Sunde, *Arch. Biochem. Biophys.*, **179**, 211 (1977).

73. H. F. DeLuca, "Vitamin D—1976," in V. H. T. James, Ed., *Endocrinology,* Excerpta Medica, Amsterdam, Vol. 2, 1977, p. 262.

74. W. M. McIndoe, "Yolk Synthesis," in D. J. Bell and B. M. Freeman, Eds., *Physiology and Biochemistry of the Domestic Fowl,* Vol. 3, Academic, New York, 1971, p. 1209.

75. E. Spanos and I. MacIntyre, *Lancet,* **1**, 840 (1977).

76. D. Fraser, S. W. Kooh, and C. R. Scriver, *Pediat. Res.*, **1**, 425 (1967).

77. E. V. McCollum, N. Simmonds, J. E. Becker, and P. G. Shipley, *J. Biol. Chem.*, **65**, 97 (1925).

78. A. Prader, R. Illig, and E. Heierli, *Helv. Paediat. Acta,* **16**, 452 (1961).

79. D. Fraser, S. W. Kooh, H. P. Kind, M. F. Holick, Y. Tanaka, and H. F. DeLuca, *New England, J. Med.*, **289**, 817 (1973).

80. B. E. Kream, M. J. L. Jose, and H. F. DeLuca, *Arch. Biochem. Biophys.*, **179**, 462 (1977).

81. J. A. Eisman and H. F. DeLuca, *Steroids,* in press (1977).

82. T. F. Williams, R. W. Winter, and C. H. Burnett, "Familial (Hereditary) Vitamin D-Resistant Rickets with Hypophosphatemia," in J. B. Stanbury, J. B. Wyngaarden, and D. S. Fredrickson, Eds., *The Metabolic Basis of Inherited Disease,* 2nd ed., McGraw-Hill, New York, 1966, p. 1179.

83. C. Arnaud, F. Glorieux, and C. Scriver, *Science,* **173,** 845 (1971).

84. F. Glorieux and C. R. Scriver, *Science,* **175,** 997 (1972).

85. E. M. Short, H. J. Binder, and L. E. Rosenberg, *Science,* **179,** 700 (1973).

86. D. Fraser and C. R. Scriver, *Am J. Clin. Nutr.,* **29,** 1315 (1976).

87. E. M. Eicher, J. L. Southard, C. R. Scriver, and F. H. Glorieux, *Proc. Nat. Acad. Sci. USA,* **73,** 4667 (1976).

88. P. J. A. O'Doherty, H. F. DeLuca, and E. M. Eicher, *Endocrinology,* in press (1977).

89. F. H. Glorieux, C. R. Scriver, T. M. Reade, H. Goldman, and A. Roseborough, *New Engl. J. Med.,* **287,** 481 (1972).

90. G. H. Hirschman, J. C. M. Chan, and H. F. DeLuca, *Pediatrics,* in press (1977).

91. H. Rassmussen, M. M. Pechet, C. Anast, J. Parks, A. Brodus, P. Bordier, and J. Lane, *New Engl. J. Med.,* in press (1977).

92. N. S. Bricker, E. Slatopolsky, E. Reiss, and L. V. Avioli, *Arch. Internal Med.,* **123,** 543 (1969).

93. A. M. Pierides, D. N. S. Kerr, H. A. Ellis, K. M. Peart, J. L. H. O'Riordan, and H. F. DeLuca, *Clin. Nephrol.,* **5,** 189 (1976).

94. J. C. M. Chan, S. B. Oldham, M. F. Holick, and H. F. DeLuca, *J.A.M.A.,* **234,** 47 (1975).

95. H. F. DeLuca, *Ann. Internal Med.,* **85,** 367 (1976).

96. S. W. Kooh, D. Fraser, H. F. DeLuca, M. F. Holick, R. E. Belsey, M. B. Clark, and T. M. Murray, *New Engl. J. Med.,* **293,** 840 (1975).

97. R. M. Neer, M. F. Holick, H. F. DeLuca, and J. T. Potts, Jr., *Metabolism,* **24,** 1403 (1975).

98. S. W. Kooh, D. Fraser, R. Toon, and H. F. DeLuca, *Lancet,* **2,** 1105 (1976).

PART 2

Proteins and Amino Acids

2

Dietary Restriction in Inborn Errors of Amino Acid Metabolism

HORST BICKEL

University Children's Hospital, Heidelberg, Germany

A few of the many inborn errors of metabolism can be treated with special diets which aim at correcting the metabolic disturbance. This chapter is limited to some errors of amino acid metabolism, in which certain foods have to be replaced by synthetic substitutes or omitted altogether. The therapeutic principle for amino acid disturbances is to give the amino acids before the enzyme block in reduced quantities, thus preventing their accumulation, which seems to be the principal damaging factor in most of these diseases. Since all natural protein sources contain the entire amino acid spectrum, special protein substitutes without the amino acids involved are essential to complete the protein requirement. This treatment was practiced for the first time in 1953, when phenylalanine-free hydrolyzates were used in phenylketonuria (1). This method then became a model for the treatment of other amino acid disturbances. Today protein hydrolyzates and synthetic amino acid mixtures are commercially available from various manufacturers.

Phenylketonuria, maple syrup urine disease, homocystinuria, supertyrosinemia, and perhaps also histidinemia can be successfully influenced with such diets. The biochemical disorder can be corrected and the clinical symptoms improved. In tyrosinosis and cystinosis trials over several years have indicated that the diets are of little or no therapeutic value. This chapter includes a more detailed account of the diets used for these amino acid disturbances.

PHENYLKETONURIA

In classical phenylketonuria (PKU), the severe deficiency of phenylalanine hydroxylase in the liver leads to an accumulation of phenylalanine, phenylpyruvic acid, and other phenolic compounds, which results in severe brain damage. It has been proven that a diet restricted in phenylalanine is successful, normalizing the excessive phenylalanine concentration in the blood and other biological fluids and thus avoiding mental retardation and cerebral convulsions (Fig. 1), (2,3). If phenylalanine loads are reintroduced into the phenylalanine-restricted diet of young patients over several days in high doses, cerebral symptoms including drowsiness, ataxia, and salivation recur.

It must be emphasized that only early treatment within the first 8 weeks of life guarantees normal development. If therapy is delayed beyond these first 2 months the results are much more equivocal and some cases show irreversible brain damage (Figs. 2 and 3) (4). Nevertheless the diet should also be initiated in older children, because limited and sometimes important improvement can still be achieved and further deterioration will be prevented (Fig. 4).

Although no definite answer can be given as to when the diet can be discontinued, it seems possible to allow a somewhat higher phenylalanine intake beyond the age of 10, probably because brain maturation

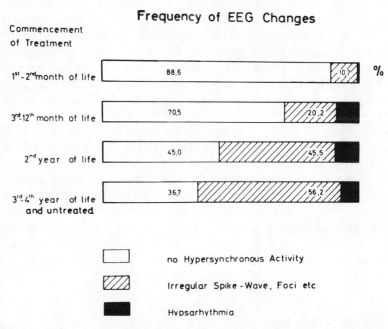

Figure 1. Frequency of EEG changes at different commencement of treatment in PKU.

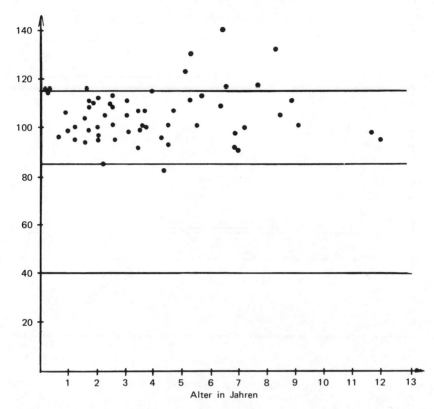

Figure 2. Latest DQ/IQ values in 60 phenylketonuric children whose treatment was started within the first 2 months of life. DQ = Development quotient, IQ = Intelligence quotient.

is then largely completed. These children are still kept under frequent clinical and biochemical supervision. Our present goal is to maintain their phenylalanine blood level below 20 mg %. I realize that the issue of when to terminate the strict diet is highly controversial. Our cautious attitude was prompted not only by the results of Cabalska in Poland (5) but also by a recent collaborative study from London and Heidelberg (6). Cabalska observed an important deterioration of mental performance in the majority of her 32 patients when the diet was terminated at 4 to 6 years of age (Fig 5). Of 85 patients from London and Heidelberg, a group of 47 patients suffered a significant decrease of their mean intelligence quotient and other negative effects when the strict diet was changed to unrestricted food intake at the age of 7 or 8.

For a phenylalanine-restricted diet, 50 to 80% of the natural protein

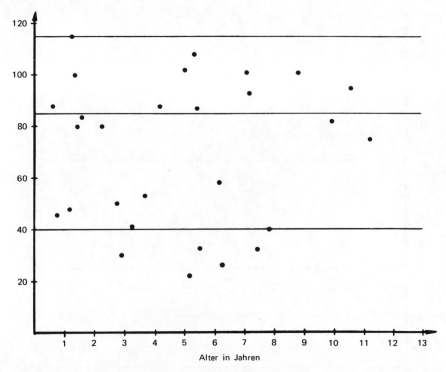

Figure 3. Latest DQ/IQ values in 28 phenylketonuric children whose treatment was delayed, starting between the third and twelfth month of life.

must be replaced by a protein preparation that contains little or no phenylalanine. The severe reduction of natural proteins in the diet may give rise to deficiencies of vitamins, minerals, and trace elements. The composition of the preparation should therefore meet all nutritional requirements (7). The most commonly used preparations are listed in Table 1 with the content of phenylalanine, other nutrients, and the necessary supplements. Two different kinds of preparations, protein hydrolyzates and synthetic amino acid mixtures, are on the market. The hydrolyzates listed are derived from casein and from ox serum protein. The protein source determines the amino acid pattern and to some extent the mineral content. Within the last few years reasonably priced synthetic amino acid mixtures have become available. With these preparations we have the choice of any desired amino acid composition.

We now have had 25 years of experience in over 200 patients with diets based on hydrolyzates. With individual treatment lasting up to 16 years, growth and gain in weight proceeded normally. There were no

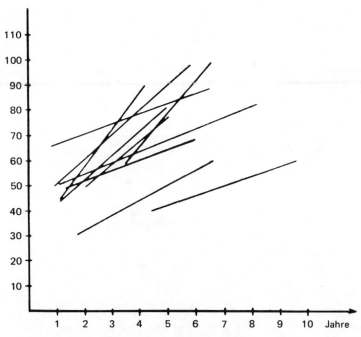

Figure 4. DQ/IQ progression of phenylketonuric children with delayed start of treatment but excellent dietary control, ensuring nearly normal phenylalanine blood levels between 2 and 4 mg %.

Table 1   Special Preparations for Phenylketonuria

	Phenyl-alanine (mg %)	Protein (g %)	Content	Necessary Supplements
Albumaid XP (SHS)	0	30	Ox serum hydrolyzate	Vitamins C, D
Cymogran (Glaxo)	10	30	Acid hydrolyzed casein	All vitamins
Lofenalac (Mead Johnson)	80	15	Enzymatic hydro-lyzed casein	—
Minafen (Trufood)	20	11, 5	Acid hydrolyzed casein	Vitamins A, C, D
Aminogran (Glaxo)	0	80	Amino acid mixture	All vitamins
PK-Aid or P-AM (SHS-Maizena)	0	75	Amino acid mixture	Vitamins C, D

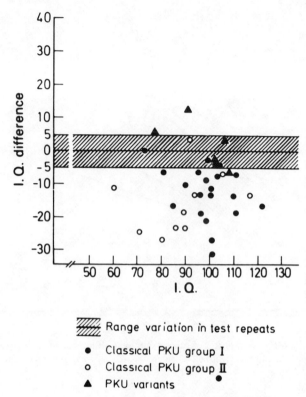

Figure 5. Differences in individual IQs of phenylketonuric (PKU) patients after discontinuation of dietary treatment at 4 to 6 years (5).

other clinical or biochemical signs of nutritional deficiencies when the intake of phenylalanine and other food components was well adjusted. Within the last 8 years we have also started to administer synthetic amino acid mixtures to a smaller group of patients.

During an initial 2-year test period 22 patients fed with synthetic amino acid mixtures have been closely observed at our hospital. A specimen diet and the conveniently smaller volume of the daily amino acid intake as contrasted to a protein hydrolyzate are shown in Table 2. Clinical supervision over the entire period of treatment with these amino acid mixtures revealed no obvious symptoms of deficiencies. Gains in growth and weight proceeded undisturbed, and no abnormalities in amino acid, protein, or mineral metabolism were found (8).

Comprehensive studies of the acid–base and electrolyte status were carried out in 64 patients on diets containing hydrolyzates and amino acid mixtures (9). Depending on the preparation, more or less marked imbalances became apparent. Metabolic acidosis was observed when the preparations contained amino acids in the form of hydrochloride salts or when the proportion of sulphur-containing amino acids was too high.

Physiologically acid production is higher in infants than in older children and adults. This explains why diets with an extra acid load resulted in marked acidosis in infants and could even cause clinical symptoms such as anorexia and vomiting. Obviously, when synthetic diets replace most of the food intake, they must be well balanced with respect not only to the amino acid pattern but also to the electrolyte composition. Table 3 lists some conclusions derived from our acid–base studies which should be considered when setting up any synthetic diet. On the basis of these conclusions, the formulas of some of these products have been improved.

For the intake of protein, carbohydrate, fat, and calories, we adhere to the international recommendations for healthy children (7). The

Table 2   Phenylalanine-Restricted Diets[a]

	Protein, (g)		
A. 4½ months, 6 kg body weight			
45 g Albumaid XP, incl. vitamins + minerals	13.5		
Natural protein			
Milk, cream	7.0	55 mg phenylalanine	per kg bw/day
Vegetables, fruits	1.8	3.7 g protein	
Cornstarch, sugar			
Oil			
Vitamin D			
B. 4 years, 17 kg body weight			
50 g Aminogran supplement	37.5		
Natural protein			
Cream	1.8		
Vegetables, potatoes, fruits	3.3	15 mg phenylalanine	per kg bw/day
Cornstarch bread	0.8	2.5 g protein	
Cornstarch, sugar			
Oil, fats			
8 g Aminogran mineral mixture + vitamins			

[a] The first patient receives a protein hydrolyzate, the second an amino acid mixture (see text).

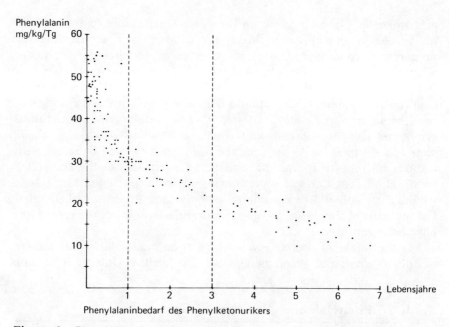

Figure 6. Phenylalanine requirement of patients with phenylketonuria at different ages, as measured by the phenylalanine intake in mg/kg/24 hours. The data were taken only from patients on a well-controlled phenylalanine-restricted diet, with phenylalanine blood levels between 1 and 4 mg % and with a satisfactory gain in weight.

Table 3   Recommendations Concerning a Balanced Acid–Base Intake in Phenylalanine-Restricted Diets

1. *Urinary sulphate* correlates well with the methionine and cystine in the diet.

   In protein hydrolyzates the methionine and cystine content must be considered.

   In synthetic amino acid mixtures methionine and cystine should not exceed 1 mM S/kg/day.

2. *Absorbed cation excess*

   Na + K should exceed Cl content.

   HCl salts of ARG, HIS, LYS should be avoided.

   Both a high intake of Ca and P and a high Ca : P ratio promote H^+ excretion.

   In synthetic amino acid mixtures P should not exceed Ca.

   Considering all factors influencing acid–base balance, renal NaE in Phe restricted preparations should lie within normal limits of 0.5 to 2 mEq/kg/day.

Table 4   Indication and Contraindication for Starting a Phenylalanine-Restricted Diet in Infants with Phenylketonuria

1. Infants with phenylalanine blood levels above 10 mg % should be treated. Phenylalanine loading tests at 6 and 12 months should confirm, the persistence of the enzyme defect. Tyrosinemia should be excluded.
2. This policy should be followed until there is unequivocal proof that phenylalanine blood levels above 10 mg %, with or without phenylpyruvic acid excretion, are harmless to the rapidly growing infantile brain.
3. Infants with phenylalanine blood levels below 10 mg % may remain untreated if normal development is ascertained by 6 monthly psychometric and EEG tests. Phenylalanine levels to be checked monthly.

tolerated phenylalanine intake is generally 200 to 400 mg/day and is relatively higher for young than for older children (Fig. 6). This small amount of phenylalanine is administered mainly in the form of vegetables, potatoes, fruits, and milk. Other foods of high protein content like meat, fish, cheese, eggs, normal bread, and cake are eliminated because of their high phenylalanine content. These nutrients have to be replaced by amino acid preparations, low protein foods, and special cornstarch products.

It is often difficult to differentiate clearly between classical phenylketonuria and other forms of milder hyperphenylalaninemia which may or may not lead to brain damage and may or may not need a phenylalanine-restricted diet. Until this differentiation is established unequivocally we adhere with only minor modifications to the indications and contraindications to start a phenylalanine-restricted diet as outlined 11 years ago at the Washington Conference on Phenylketonuria (Table 4) (10).

MAPLE SYRUP URINE DISEASE

It is much more difficult to treat maple syrup urine disease successfully than phenylketonuria. This disorder involves three essential amino acids: leucine, isoleucine, and valine. The clinical signs of the syndrome, the peculiar maple syrup odor, opisthotonus, asphyxia, and convulsions, manifest themselves during the first days of life on a normal milk formula. Without treatment, brain damage rapidly progresses, leading to cerebral demyelination and death within the first weeks or months of life (Figs. 7 and 8). Therapy should therefore be initiated at the earliest possible moment.

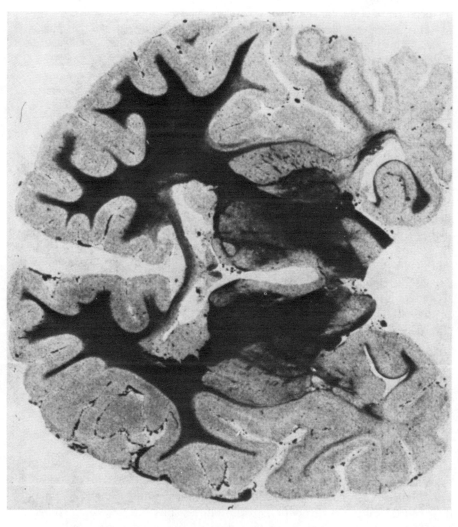

Figure 7. Brain section of a treated patient with maple syrup urine disease aged 4 months. Staining of the myelin sheets shows normal myelogenesis.

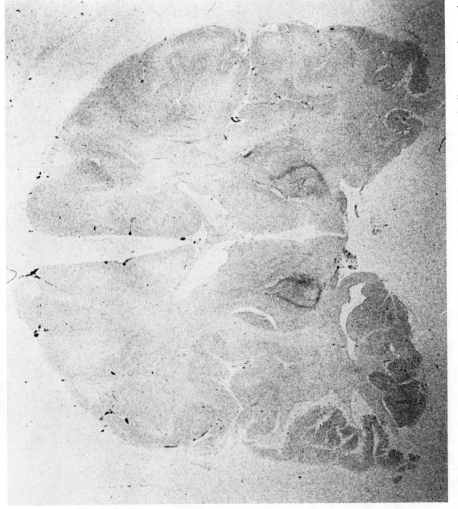

Figure 8. In an untreated patient of the same age staining fails to show practically any myelogenesis.

Table 5   Important Considerations for the Treatment of the Acute Neonatal Phase in Maple Syrup Urine Disease (MSUD)

1. Appropriate i.v. therapy to correct acidosis and electrolyte imbalances.
2. Ventilatory assistance and anticonvulsant therapy if necessary.
3. Rapid elimination of branched-chain amino and keto acids by
   a. multiple exchange transfusions
   b; peritoneal dialysis.
4. High calorie and amino acid intake excluding branched-chain amino acids.

To master the acute neonatal phase of maple syrup disease, which can be highly dramatic, series of multiple exchange transfusions or peritoneal dialysis may be life-saving (Table 5). Furthermore, the findings in three recent patients convinced us that—besides multiple exchange transfusions—high caloric intake of 155 to 175 cal/kg body weight daily is necessary to lower the plasma concentration of the branched-chain amino acids to almost normal levels. As long as this caloric intake was not provided to our patients, further exchange transfusions failed to reduce the plasma leucine concentration below 15 mg/100 ml. A high caloric intake seems in this phase of the disease necessary to prevent the breakdown of endogenous protein (Fig. 9) (11).

Table 6 shows a diet formula for a 7-month-old patient. This diet is largely synthetic, consisting mainly of an amino acid mixture free of the branched-chain amino acids but including vitamins and minerals (72). Carbohydrates and fats are administered in their pure form. The diet contains only traces of natural protein, usually in the form of whey, milk, and yeast to meet any possible deficiencies that may result from such a synthetic diet. Twelve years ago we observed two patients who died within their first year from nutritional deficiencies of unknown origin (13). Since then, however, a number of patients could be kept alive with the aid of such diets. Height and weight lie in the lower normal range, and there is only slight mental retardation. One of the difficulties of treatment is the constant fluctuation in the tolerance for the three amino acids involved, which requires frequent plasma aminograms. Infections lead to rapid metabolic imbalances (Fig. 10).

It is not yet known how long this diet must be continued and if one will ever be able to relax or even stop it. Biochemical monitoring certainly becomes easier with advancing age of the patient.

Very rarely one may encounter a patient with the mild, intermittent form of the disease who may develop quite normally, being threatened only occasionally during mild infections or longer episodes by severe attacks of ketotic vomiting and drowsiness, and exhibiting only then the

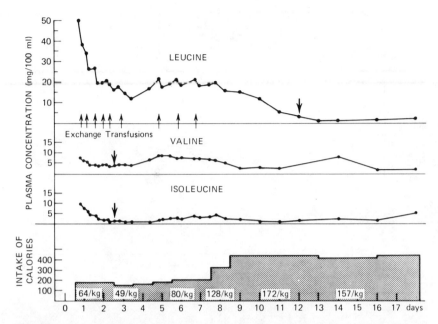

Figure 9. Treatment and biochemical control of a newborn infant with maple syrup urine disease.

↑ = blood exchange transfusion. ↓ = introduction of the individual branched-chain amino acid to the diet. For details see text.

Table 6 Diet Formula for a 7-Month-Old Patient with MSUD; Body Weight 6.4 kg

	Protein (g)		
28 g L-amino acid mixture, incl. vitamins + minerals	20		
Natural protein			
500 g whey			
20 g cow's milk	2.7	55 mg leucine	
2 g dry yeast		25 mg isoleucine	per kg bw/day
30 g potatoes		40 mg valine	
		3.6 g protein	
30 g corn oil			
20 g corn starch			
90 g dextrose			
162 mg leucine			
93 mg valine			

47

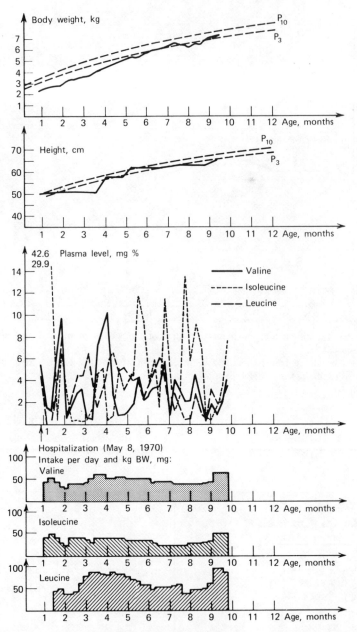

Figure 10. The course of the disease of a patient with maple syrup urine disease during the first year of life, showing the increments in body weight and leucine (mg/kg/day). Note the remarkable variation of the plasma levels of the branched-chain amino acids despite their frequent monitoring by plasma column chromatography and consequent dietary adjustment.

typical maple syrup smell. Protein restriction and fluid, electrolyte, and glucose infusions generally suffice to bring the situation under control.

HOMOCYSTINURIA

Homocystinuria is clinically characterized by a Marfan-like syndrome with skeletal changes and ectopy of the lens, mental retardation, and thromboembolic complications, often resulting in the death of these patients. The biochemical disturbance involves the metabolism of methionine. Because of a deficiency of cystathionine synthetase in the liver, methionine is not transformed to cystine. Methionine, homocystine, and mixed disulfides accumulate in blood and urine (for details see (14)).

In approximately half of these patients, a biochemical normalization occurs after treatment with large amounts of pyridoxine, the cofactor of cystathionine synthetase. This group of patients shows some rest activity of the enzyme, which is activated by pyridoxine. Patients without any enzyme activity do not respond to pyridoxine supplementation. In these cases one can achieve biochemical normalization by restricting methionine intake. This again means that the diet has to be complemented with special preparations low in or free of methionine. Further additions include choline as a methyl group donor, and cystine, which becomes an essential amino acid in this disease. A specimen diet is given in Table 7. Although some promising results have been achieved, an evaluation of this treatment is still difficult because the natural course of the disease is chronic, progressing only slowly over many years.

Table 7   Diet Formula for a 7-Year-Old Patient with Homocystinuria; Body Weight 28 kg

	Protein (g)		
100 g Albumaid X Met., incl. vitamins + minerals	30 ⎫		
Natural protein			
Milk	6 ⎬	17 mg methionine ⎫	
Eggs	6	1.8 g protein	
Vegetables, potatoes, fruits	6	3.3 g fat ⎬ per kg bw/day	
Cornstarch products	2 ⎭	12 g carbohydrate	
		90 calories ⎭	
Carbohydrates, fats	⎫		
Choline + cystine	⎬		

HISTIDINEMIA

In histidinemia the enzyme defect blocks the transformation of histidine into urocanic acid, which leads to brain damage in an unknown percentage of the patients (15,16). Though the brain damage is not as severe as and much less frequent than in phenylketonuria, we agree with Thalhammer that a prophylactic histidine-restricted diet should be introduced within the first months of life. Other well-informed authors do not consider that the need for such an incisive therapy is proven and allow their patients a normal food intake without histidine restriction. A histidine-restricted menu differs from the former diets only in the composition of the amino acid preparation, which is free of histidine. As to the effectiveness of this diet, it is too early to draw any definite conclusions. Thalhammer, who has the most experience in Europe, claims that so far his patients have developed normally on the diet. One of his infant patients deteriorated when taken off the diet by its mother (17).

TYROSINEMIAS

Of the different tyrosinemias only two will be discussed; namely, tyrosinemia type I, also called tyrosinosis by European authors, and tyrosinemia type II. In tyrosinosis the metabolic disorder is still obscure. Most authors believe that tyrosinemia and, in some cases methioninemia, are secondary phenomena of a liver disease of unknown origin. For this reason the rationale of dietary treatment with restriction of phenylalanine and tyrosine (Table 8) has become questionable. In our own experience healing of rickets, normalization of phosphate in serum, and increased tubular phosphate reabsorption were seen during dietary tyrosine restriction, but there was no direct influence on other symptoms such as liver dysfunction and thrombocytopenia (18). Halvorsen followed four Norwegian patients for 5 to 10 years; the improvements in renal phosphate reabsorption, amino aciduria, rickets, and neuromuscular functions were greater in the two patients on dietary treatment than in the two patients treated solely with vitamin D. There was no improvement of liver function in any of these patients (19).

More rewarding is the dietary therapy of type II tyrosinemia, also called supertyrosinemia or tyrosinemia with keratitis and palmoplantar keratosis. This rare disease is caused by a hereditary tyrosine aminotransferase defect, which leads to a heavy accumulation of tyrosine and some of its metabolites in blood, urine, and other biological fluids (Fig. 11). The leading clinical symptoms are a very painful keratitis of the

Table 8   Diet Formula for a 1.9-Year-Old Patient with Tyrosinosis; Body Weight 10 kg

	Protein (g)	
35 g phenylalanine + tyrosine-free amino acid mixture incl. vitamins + minerals	25.5	
Natural protein:		
200 g cow's milk ⎫ 80 g double cream ⎭	8.0	50 mg tyrosine ⎫ 50 mg phenylalanine ⎬ kg/bw/day 3.6 g protein ⎭
50 g potatoes ⎫ 150 g carrots ⎬ 100 g bananas ⎭	3.0	
cornstarch products 100 g dextrose 20 g corn oil		

eyes, which practically blinds the child, painful plantar and palmar keratosis of the skin, and mental retardation (20,21). None of these symptoms has been regularly present in more than 20 cases described so far, although the ocular lesion seems to be first in frequency and has even been observed in a 3-week-old infant by Halvorsen (22). In contrast to tyrosinosis, liver and kidney functions are normal. Under a tyrosine-restricted diet, the blinding keratitis and the skin lesions heal within days or weeks, and damage to the brain can possibly be prevented. The excellent effect of this therapy stresses the importance of an early diagnosis, before mental retardation has occurred.

CYSTINOSIS

In cystinosis, the last disorder of amino acid metabolism to be discussed, dietetic treatment is probably ineffective. The enzyme defect is still unknown. Cystine is stored intracellularly in the lysosomes. Proximal tubular damage leads to a Fanconi syndrome with dwarfism and vitamin D-resistant rickets. At a later stage, complex renal failure develops and finally death occurs due to uremia, generally before puberty is reached.

During the last 10 years attempts have been made to influence the natural course of cystinosis by giving a diet restricted in cystine and

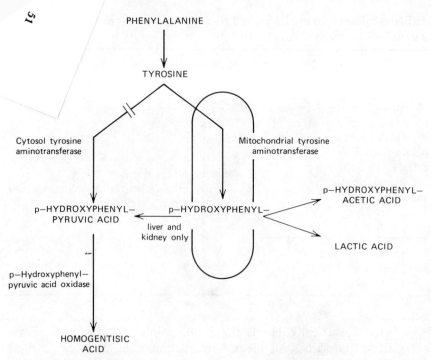

Figure 11. Position of the cytosol tyrosine aminotransferase defect in type II tyrosinemia.

methionine. The effect of this treatment has been evaluated in 21 patients from Heidelberg and other European pediatric centers (23). Unfortunately the course of the disease was not influenced by the diet but remained progressive. It remains to be seen if newer therapeutic approaches to this deleterious disease will prove more successful, such as the use of high doses of ascorbic acid or the more powerful but also more toxic cysteamine for intracellular cystine depletion.

There is some reason to believe that cystine storage is not the actual pathogenetic factor of this disease. If this were true, then the depletion of cystine stores by diet or drugs would not be the primary therapeutic goal.

Dietary treatment of inborn errors of amino acid metabolism is a secondary, cumbersome way to correct the metabolic disturbance. The direct approach of enzyme replacement is not yet available, but may well become a preferable possibility in the future management of these patients.

REFERENCES

1. H. Bickel, J. Gerrard and E. M. Hickmans, *Lancet,* **2,** 312 (1953).
2. H. Bickel and S. Kaiser-Grubel, *Dtsch. med. Wschr.* **96,** 1415 (1971).
3. A. Lütcke, in H. Bickel, F. P. Hudson, and L. I. Woolf, Eds., *Phenylketonuria,* Thieme, Stuttgart, 1971, p. 269.
4. E. Schmid-Rüter and S. Grubel-Kaiser, *Mschr. Kinderheilk.,* **125,** 479 (1977).
5. B. Cabalska, B. Prindull, W. Schröter, and J. M. Yoffey, *Eur. J. Pediat.,* **126,** 253 (1977).
6. I. Smith, M. Lobascher, J. Stevenson, O. H. Wolff, H. Schmidt, S. Grubel-Kaiser, and H. Bickel, 1978, in preparation.
7. H. Bickel, H. Schmidt, and L. Schürrle, Bibl. "Nutr. Diet.," Karger, Basel, 1973, p. 181.
8. P. Lutz, H. Schmidt, L. Schürrle, and H. Bickel, *Proceed. XIII International Pediatric Congress,* Vienna, 1971, vol. V/1, p. 41.
9. F. Manz, H. Schmidt, K. Schärer, and H. Bickel, *Ped. Res.,* 1978 (in press).
10. H. Bickel, in J. A. Anderson and K. F. Swaiman, Eds., *Phenylketonuria and Allied Metabolic Diseases.* Proceed of a Conf., Washington, D.C., April 6–8, 1966. U.S. Dept. HEW, U.S. Govt. Printing Office, Washington D.C., 1967.
11. G. Hammersen, L. Wille, H. Schmidt, P. Lutz and H. Bickel, *Eur. J. Pediat.,* 1978 (in press).
12. S. E. Snyderman, in Raines, Ed., *The Treatment of Inherited Metabolic Disease,* Medical and Technical Publishing Co., Lancaster, 1975, p. 71.
13. F. Linneweh and U. Willenbockel, *Mschr. Kinderheilk.,* **113,** 420 (1965).
14. L. D. Fleisher and G. E. Gaull, in H. Bickel, Ed., *Congenital and Acquired Diseases of Amino Acid Metabolism,* Clinics in Endocrinology and Metabolism, Vol. 3, No. 1, Saunders, London, 1974, p. 37.
15. H. L. Levy, V. E. Shih, P. M. Madigan, *New Engl. J. Med.,* **291,** 1214 (1974).
16. T. Arakawa, in H. Bickel, Ed., *Clinics in Endocrinology and Metabolism,* Saunders, London, 1974, p. 17.
17. O. Thalhammer, personal communication.
18. W. Nützenadel, P. Lutz, and H. Bickel, *Z. Kinderheilk.,* **113,** 193 (1972).
19. S. Halvorsen and L. R. Gjessing, in H. Bickel, F. P. Hudson, and L. I. Woolf, Eds., *Phenylketonuria and some other Inborn Errors of Amino Acid Metabolism,* Thieme, Stuttgart, 1971, p. 301.
20. L. A. Goldsmith, E. Kang, D. C. Bienfang, K. Jimbow, P. Gerald, and H. P. Baden, *J. Pediatr.,* **83,** 798 (1973).
21. L. R. Garibaldi, F. Siliato, I. Martini, M. R. Scarsi, and C. Romano. *Helv. paediat. Acta,* **32,** 173 (1977).
22. S. Halvorsen and L. Skelkvale, *Ped. Res.,* **11,** 1017 (1977).
23. H. Bickel, P. Lutz, and H. Schmidt, in J. D. Schulman, *Cystinosis.* U.S. DHEW Publ. No. (NIH) 72–249, U.S. Govt. Printing Office, Washington, D.C., p. 199.

3

Use of Cofactors in Inborn Errors of Amino Acid Metabolism

LEON E. ROSENBERG, M.D.

Yale University School of Medicine, New Haven, Connecticut

The use of nutritional management, as outlined in the previous chapters, was the first form of therapy attempted in inborn errors of metabolism.

This chapter deals with the second mode of therapy that has been used during recent years, namely, the use of vitamin cofactors in the treatment of inborn errors of amino acid metabolism. This mode of therapy arose as a consequence of a series of now classic clinical observations.

The first was a case described by Dr. Hunt and his associates at Philadelphia Children's Hospital. It began in 1954 with the birth of a baby girl who began having major epileptic seizures on the second day of life after an uneventful pregnancy and delivery and died of uncontrollable seizures on the third day of life. A few years later a second female infant was born to the same mother. She was noted to be very jittery at birth and she also began having seizures on the fifth day of life. She was treated very quickly with barbiturates, with magnesium sulfate, and with calcium gluconate and failed to respond. As part of a general supportive therapy, this little girl was given large amounts of a multivitamin preparation containing all of the water-soluble B vitamins and vitamin C and her seizures stopped abruptly. During the next 3 weeks this cyclic course of seizures abruptly halted by the water-soluble vitamin preparation was reproduced and convinced the clinicians that this was, in fact, a cause and effect relationship. Then the individual vitamins in the mixture were administered one at a time and it became clear that vitamin B_6 (pyridoxine) and only vitamin B_6 was the agent responsible for controlling the seizure disorder. The child was then placed on physiologic amounts of pyridoxine but the seizures recurred, and only when the child was given somewhere between 5 and 20 times the usual physiologic doses was the seizure disorder regulated. The features, then, of this case were the familial nature of the seizures and the supraphysiologic requirement for a single water-soluble vitamin. This child, or these children, were called cases of "vitamin B_6-dependent seizure disorder." Many more children with a similar clinical constellation have been described subsequently, and although we still do not know the biochemical basis for this kind of pyridoxine responsiveness, these children present the hallmark of the disorders that I want to discuss.

In the past several years it has become clear that a number of other enzymatic disturbances of amino acid metabolism will respond to supraphysiologic amounts of pyridoxine and in many of those instances we understand the biochemical basis for the disorder much better than we do in classic pyridoxine-responsive seizures.

The second major series of clinical observations that I shall describe concerns vitamin B_{12} responsiveness. These observations began in our own laboratory in 1968 when a child was admitted at age 9 months in a comatose state. He was found to have a blood pH lower than 7 and an undetectable plasma-bicarbonate concentration. After bicarbonate therapy restored his blood pH to values consistent with prolonged life, a long series of metabolic investigations were undertaken. The data revealed that this child was excreting in his urine about 1500 times as much of a simple dicarboxylic acid, called methylamalonic acid, as is excreted in normal individuals. In addition, parenteral administration of huge doses of vitamin B_{12} to this child caused a marked reduction in the excretion of methylmalonic acid. I should point out that there was a rationale for the use of vitamin B_{12} in this case, since it was known that the reaction by which methylmalonate is converted to succinate is catalyzed by an enzyme which requires a vitamin B_{12} cofactor, adenosylcobalamin or adenosyl-B_{12}. Hence this was an example of vitamin B_{12} responsiveness based on a sound chemical rationale. However, there was more than chemical responsiveness in this situation for we could mitigate the toxic effect of valine, a precursor of methylmalonate, by loading the child with vitamin B_{12}. Not only was the excretion of methylmalonate following valine administration markedly reduced when the child was receiving B_{12} supplements but there was a reduction in the tendency to develop ketoacidosis. This child then was treated with one thousand times as much vitamin B_{12} as any of us supposedly requires, for a number of years. He is now 11 years old, lives in Florida, is a healthy and active boy, and an honor roll student.

He no longer takes vitamin B_{12}, the family having decided a few years ago that they simply were not going to continue that form of therapy. He excretes huge amounts of methylmalonic acid in his urine and yet he has had no recent disturbance of acid–base balance.

I have discussed these two particular clinical situations in some detail because they epitomize the features of the vitamin-responsive disorders of amino acid metabolism that I shall now review.

The common features of these patients, then, were the early onset of life-threatening symptoms and signs, a dramatic response to supra-physiologic amounts of a single vitamin, and evidence for Mendelian inheritance implying the involvement of mutations at a single genetic locus. In the past 10 years this field has evolved in a number of ways. First, a large number of other vitamin-responsive inherited metabolic disorders of amino acid metabolism have been described. Second, the description of such children has spurred the investigation of mechanisms of genetic control of vitamin metabolism and of the role of vitamins as cofactors in a number of biochemical systems. And, finally, these children have led to the realization that a small number of children have unique vitamin requirements which, if recognized, make the difference between a productive life and a failed existence. Let me turn to the panorama of these disorders as we currently understand them.

There are approximately 20 different metabolic disorders of amino acid metabolism which meet the three essential criteria for inclusion in this discussion. First, a clear genetic etiology; second, a characteristic clinical or biochemical phenotype; and third, unequivocal chemical or clinical responsiveness or both to a supraphysiologic amount or an ex-traphysiologic route of administration of a single vitamin. I prefer to call these disorders "vitamin-responsive" diseases rather than "vitamin-dependent" ones because the term vitamin dependency seems to produce some confusion.

Table 1 lists these conditions according to the vitamin that is required to treat them. They fall into six different categories. The largest number of disorders described to date are those involving pyridoxine responsive-ness. In each of the conditions involving pyridoxine responsiveness, the defect appears to be due to a primary abnormality of a single pyridoxal-phosphate-dependent apoenzyme such that cofactor supplementation restores enzymatic activity at least toward normal. The second major group of disorders involve defects in vitamin B_{12} metabolism. All of the disorders classified here are rare. Some have been reported in only one or two families. All except pyridoxine-responsive hypochromic anemia appear to be inherited as autosomal recessive traits, implying a double dose of a single mutant gene. The hypochromic anemia that responds to

Table 1   Vitamin-Responsive Inherited Metabolic Diseases

Thiamine (vitamin B_1)
  Branched-chain ketoaciduria
  Cerebellar ataxia
  Lacticacidosis
  Megaloblastic anemia
Pyridoxine (vitamin B_6)
  Cystathioninuria
  Homocystinuria
  Hypochromic anemia
  Infantile convulsions
  Oxalosis
  Xanthurenic aciduria
Cobalamin (vitamin B_{12})
  Ileal transport defect
  Inert intrinsic factor
  Intrinsic factor deficiency
  Methylmalonicacidemia
  Methylmalonicacidemia and
    homocystinuria
  Transcobalamin II deficiency

Folic acid
  Formiminotransferase deficiency
  Homocystinuria and hypometh-
    ioninemia
  Intestinal malabsorption
  Megaloblastic anemia
Biotin
  β-Methylcrotonylglycinuria
  Propionicacidemia
Nicotinamide
  Hartnup disease

pyridoxine is known to be X-linked. Nearly all of these conditions have been described in infants or young children, many in the neonatal period. It would be impossible to try to survey each of these disorders but let me simply point out that three major clinical phenotypes have emerged in these children that we must think about if we are going to recognize children with these conditions. More than half of the disorders on this list alter central nervous system development, leading to either seizures or ataxia or mental retardation or behavioral aberrations. Hence neonates or young infants with major neurologic disorders of ill-defined etiology must be considered candidates for disorders shown on this list. An almost equal number of disorders on this list present with metabolic acidosis or ketosis, and again, therefore, an infant with unexplained disturbances of acid–base balance must be considered a candidate for a vitamin-responsive disease. And, finally, half a dozen conditions here manifest anemia as a major presenting sign.

Let us very briefly examine the biochemical basis for these vitamin-responsive disorders. We now recognize two general classes of mutations: those that involve vitamin metabolism per se, and those in which vitamin metabolism appears to be normal but in which the genetic defect involves a specific apoenzyme that needs a vitamin cofactor for normal activity. It has already been noted that all of the pyridoxine-responsive disorders are due to specific apoenzyme defects and not to disorders of pyridoxine metabolism. Let me now concentrate on disorders of vitamin B_{12} or cobalamin metabolism because it is in this group that we now recognize diseases due, in some instances, to defective vitamin metabolism and, in others, to defective apoproteins that require vitamin cofactors. What do we know about genetic control of vitamin metabolism, particularly of water-soluble vitamins that act as enzymatic cofactors? Although by definition the human organism has lost the ability to make vitamins, we have retained a very complex and highly regulated system for the utilization of vitamins at all levels. Thus normal vitamin utilization depends on a number of metabolic events that are under genetic control (Fig. 1).

Regulation of vitamin metabolism could take place at the level of intestinal absorption, of plasma transport, of cellular entry, of intracellular compartmentation of the vitamin, of conversion of a vitamin precursor to its active coenzyme form, and finally at the level of formation of an active holoenzyme by attachment of the vitamin cofactor to the apoprotein which requires it. In a theoretical sense then, one can imagine that if there are six different steps for the normal utilization of any particular vitamin, there must be six different kinds of proteins and, hence, six different genetic loci required for normal metabolism of any single vitamin species. If this scheme is correct, we can then make some predictions

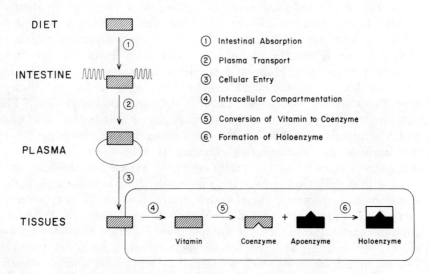

Figure 1. Steps required for normal vitamin utilization by human tissues. Each step is under genetic control and is subject to mutation.

about inherited variation in vitamin metabolism. For instance, we can predict that mutations might be expected to alter each of the proteins and, hence, each of the steps involved; that for a given vitamin, mutations at different steps will produce very different biochemical consequences. Hence if there is a genetic defect in intestinal absorption, one would expect that all reactions inside the cell that depend on that vitamin would be impaired. On the other hand, if a vitamin normally is used in the cell in more than one way, or in more than one coenzyme form, defects at the level of coenzyme synthesis might impair only a single reaction rather than multiple ones. And, finally, one would predict that abnormalities in a specific apoprotein ought to be biochemically distinct and leave other reactions catalyzed by the same vitamin unimpaired. We can go further in such predictions and expect that mutations of any one of these steps which lead to the complete absence or complete deficiency of activity of a particular protein would not be expected to respond to any amount of vitamin supplement unless we circumvent the block by altering the route of administration. If the mutations involved are "leaky," that is, if there is some residual activity, then administration of supraphysiologic amounts of vitamin may allow for enhanced residual activity according to mass action principles. Let us examine how this theoretical framework fits with known vitamin-responsive disorders by discussing in more detail vitamin B_{12}-responsive or cobalamin-responsive conditions.

Vitamin B_{12} is required normally in minute amounts, only about 1 μg/day being required. The vitamin is synthesized only by microorganisms and man must derive his dietary needs from intake mainly of animal tissues where the vitamin is stored or in lesser amounts from particular vegetables. Humans have devised, retained, or developed a very complex mechanism for utilization of the ingested vitamin. Absorption of vitamin B_{12} requires a number of different binding proteins. The first, in the stomach, called the intrinsic factor, binds the cobalamin which is consumed in the diet, and carries it to the small intestine where the intrinsic factor–cobalamin complex is split. The cobalamin is transported actively by a specific receptor system in the intestinal mucosa into the blood, where it again binds to various proteins called transcobalamin proteins, one of which, transcobalamin II, is required to carry the vitamin to tissues and to enhance its uptake by cells. When the vitamin reaches the tissues, we know a good bit more about the nature of the cell biology and biochemistry. We now understand that the vitamin complexed to its transcobalamin carrier protein binds to specific cell surface receptors and the complex is taken into the cell by adsorptive endocytosis. The endocytotic vesicle fuses with primary lysosomes, yielding secondary lysosomes in which the transcobalamin protein is split and the vitamin is released into the cytoplasm. There it is used to form methylcobalamin, which is the coenzyme for a reaction catalyzed by methionine synthetase (Fig. 2). This reaction also requires methyltetrahydrofolate as a cosubstrate. Alternatively, the cytosolic vitamin may gain entrance to the mitochondrial matrix where, via a very complex series of enzymatically catalyzed reactions, the nucleus of the vitamin is first reduced by reductase enzymes and then acted upon by an adenosyltransferase to form adenosylcobalamin, the specific active cofactor needed by the mutase system. From this panorama it is apparent that if you have intestinal binding proteins, specific ileal receptors, transcobalamins in the blood, receptor systems at the cell membrane, and reductases and adenosyltransferases, there are a number of sites at which potential mutations could lead to imparied vitamin metabolism.

We now are beginning to recognize a large number of inborn errors of vitamin B_{12} metabolism at all of these various levels of tissue organization. We know of specific abnormalities in intrinsic factor or in the ileal transport system which lead to defective intestinal absorption of the vitamin and, importantly, which can be completely circumvented in a therapeutic sense simply by giving physiologic amounts of the vitamin parenterally. We also know that there are inherited abnormalities that affect the plasma transport of the vitamin; deficiencies of each of the two major transcobalamin species; and disorders of coenzyme biosynthesis in which the reductase or adenosyltransferase is impaired. In these situations the question of whether the affected child will be responsive to increased amounts of the vitamin will depend on the nature of the mutation, on the severity of the mutation, and on the significance of the particular enzymatic deficiency in question. At the present time there

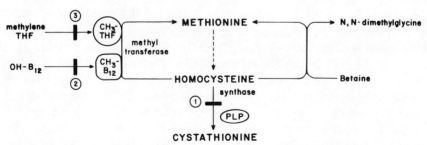

Figure 2. Partial pathway of sulfur amino acid metabolism localizing the three vitamin-responsive homocystinurias. 1: Pyridoxine-responsive cystathionine synthase deficiency. 2: B_{12}-responsive defect in methyl-B_{12} synthesis. 3: Folate-responsive N^5,N^{10}-methylenetetrahydrofolate reductase deficiency. PLP = *pyridoxal-5′*-phosphate; OH-B_{12} = hydroxocobalamin; THF = tetrahydrofolate.

are four known defects in tissue utilization of the vitamin, two of which almost certainly affect cytosolic reactions and which impair the ability to synthesize both cobalamin cofactors. Two others involve intramitochondrial enzymes because they impair the synthesis only of adenosylcobalamin. In each of these four defects of cobalamin metabolism, increased amounts of the vitamin precursor have been shown to be corrective in some infants. Thus, it is apparent that each of these different mutations must be leaky in the sense that massive amounts of precursor may restore some activity of the entire pathway.

What is the clinical significance of these observations? Vitamin supplements should be tried on any child with methylmalonic acidemia because a short course of high dose vitamin therapy of this sort cannot be harmful and may be very advantageous for children like the boy described earlier. But this kind of pathway study has led to more than just the ability to treat the affected children. Because most of these studies have been carried out with cultured cells, it has become possible to diagnose such disorders of vitamin B_{12} metabolism prenatally and, hence, to allow families to prepare for the care of an infant who is going to require vitamin B_{12} supplementation from birth on. Finally, there is a unique observation, made by Dr. Mary Ampola from Boston and Dr. Maurice Mahoney from Yale, which suggests that the knowledge of such vitamin B_{12}-responsive disorders may have an impact on fetal therapy as well as postnatal therapy. In one woman known to be carrying a fetus affected with vitamin B_{12}-responsive methylmalonic acidemia, methylmalonate excretion in her urine rose after midpregnancy. When she was given very large amounts of either oral or parenteral vitamin B_{12}, there was a distinct fall in her urinary methylmalonate excretion. We know that these urinary findings reflected modification of the metabolism of her affected fetus because a heterozygous mother carrying an unaffected fetus does not show excessive methylmalonate excretion. Thus these data demonstrate that excessive excretion of methylmalonate by a heterozygous mother is a means of diagnosing the disease prenatally. The response to the B_{12} supplements suggests that one has modified the metabolism of the fetus by the transplacental passage of vitamin administered to the mother. Is there any reason to believe that such affected fetuses may be damaged in utero; that is, that the maternal circulation may not be completely protective in a metabolic sense? We have no good answer to that question but the observed chemical response suggests that there is at least reason to probe the question further.

Thus far I have discussed beneficial effects of individual vitamins. However, it is important to realize that when we use vitamins in huge amounts, they may not any longer be acting simply as cofactors. They are now being presented to the body in pharmacologic doses and, therefore, we must be concerned about side effects. We have unpublished evidence, for example, that hydroxocobalamin (vitamin B_{12}) is a rather effective competitive inhibitor of the mutase enzyme which its cofactor, adenosylcobalamin, is a cofactor for. Thus one can imagine that a huge excess of the vitamin might impair the very reaction that one is trying to stimulate. I have recently been told of a child with methylmalonic acidemia in whom there is some reason to believe that the massive amounts of vitamin B_{12} which were given appropriately to try to correct the metabolic abnormality may, in fact, have made the abnormality worse by increasing the amount of precursor vitamin to values 10,000 or even 100,000 times normal in the cells of that particular child.

Where, then, are we with these vitamin-responsive disorders? First, we are identifying an increasing number of such conditions and we are learning more about the mechanism of some of them. We must continue to look for other mechanisms of responsiveness, such as vitamin activation of alternative pathways of metabolism. For instance, there are now biochemical data suggesting that huge amounts of pyridoxal phosphate may, by Schiff base formation, alter enzymes that do not require pyridoxal phosphate as cofactor. Second, we must continue to look for opportunities to utilize this information for the treatment of children who need such physiologic supplementation. But I am concerned about misusing the information obtained in studying and treating children with vitamin-responsive disorders through overextrapolation. The work that I have been discussing has been seized upon by proponents of megavitamin therapy as a rationale for the use of vitamins in the treatment of the common cold, or impotence, or schizophrenia, or autism, or mental retardation, or even cancer. Let me suggest that because a few patients with specific genetic disorders respond to supplements of a single vitamin, it in no way follows that all individuals with a myriad of complex disorders will benefit from supplements of many vitamins. Yet that is the extrapolation which I think some people are prepared to make. We know that some vitamins are toxic if ingested in large enough amounts. For fat-soluble vitamins that evidence is strong; for water-soluble vitamins, the evidence is increasing. I believe that when compounds designed for trace use are ingested in huge quantities, they will behave as any other pharmacologic agent with attendant side effects. Until that belief has been carefully and vigorously tested, the indiscriminant use of megadoses of vitamins seems both unwise and unwarranted.

Thus there are two sides to the vitamin-responsive metabolic disease story. I think the second side is as important as the first. I remain hopeful that, for the benefit of patients, astute clinicians, nutritionists, and investigators will assemble the new information that is required and will reconcile the conflicting claims that are being made.

REFERENCES

1. S. H. Mudd, *Fed. Proc.*, **30,** 970 (1971).
2. L. E. Rosenberg, in *Brain Dysfunction in Metabolic Disorders,* F. Plum, ed., Raven, New York, 1974, pp. 263–72.
3. C. R. Scriver and L. E. Rosenberg, in *Amino Acid Metabolism and Its Disorders,* Saunders, Philadelphia, 1973, pp. 453–78.
4. L. E. Rosenberg, in *Advances in Human Genetics,* Vol. 6, H. Harris and K. Hirschhorn, eds., Plenum, New York, 1976, pp. 1–74.
5. L. E. Rosenberg, in J. B. Stanbury, J. B. Wyngaarden, and D. S. Fredrickson, eds., *The Metabolic Basis of Inherited Disease,* 4th ed., McGraw-Hill, New York, 1978, pp. 411–29.

4

Use of Keto Acids in Inborn Errors of Urea Synthesis

SAUL BRUSILOW

Children's Medical & Surgical Center, Johns Hopkins University Hospital, Baltimore, Maryland

MARK BATSHAW

Department of Pediatrics, Johns Hopkins University Hospital, and John F. Kennedy Institute, Baltimore, Maryland

and

MACKENZIE WALSER

Department of Pharmacology & Experimental Therapeutics, Johns Hopkins Hospital, Baltimore, Maryland

Inborn errors of urea cycle enzymes occur at an estimated frequency of 1 in every 30,000 live births. While this is a rather low rate of occurrence, the number of patients recognized to have these disorders is probably even lower because most of these infants die at birth or soon thereafter. Therapy has traditionally consisted of protein restriction and, more recently, the use of supplements of essential amino acids. Various other substances have also been tried in individual disorders of this class, without clear-cut benefit in preventing death or mental retardation.

In collaboration with others, we have now treated 14 children with urea cycle enzymopathies with a low protein diet supplemented with the

These studies were supported by U.S.P.H.S Grants # AM18020, HD1134 and The Kennedy Foundation.

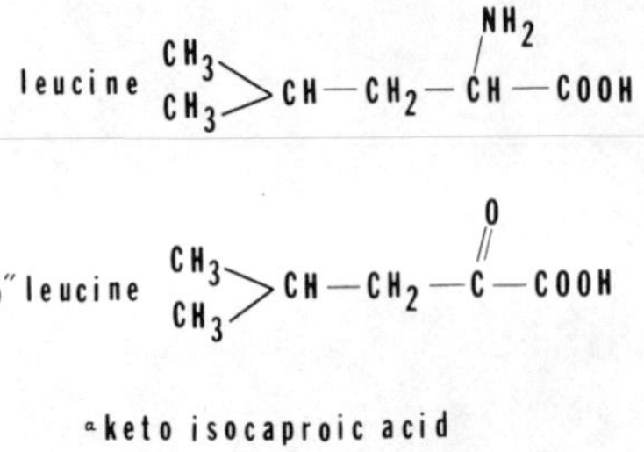

leucine $\begin{matrix} CH_3 \\ CH_3 \end{matrix}>CH-CH_2-\overset{\overset{NH_2}{|}}{CH}-COOH$

"keto" leucine $\begin{matrix} CH_3 \\ CH_3 \end{matrix}>CH-CH_2-\overset{\overset{O}{\parallel}}{C}-COOH$

α-keto isocaproic acid

Figure 1. Leucine compared to its ketone analog, α-ketoisocaproic acid.

nitrogen-free analogs of valine, leucine, isoleucine, methionine, phenylalanine, plus the remaining essential amino acids and arginine.

Figure 1 shows an example of the nitrogen-free analog of leucine, α-ketoisocaproic acid, compared to leucine itself. The only difference is the substitution of a ketone group for the amino group. When hydroxy analogs are used a hydroxyl group replaces the amino group.

A simplified scheme for the disposal of waste nitrogen and the pathway whereby it may be altered by the keto analogs is shown in Figure 2. The amino group of a nonessential amino acid is ultimately transaminated to glutamate, which is deaminated by glutamate dehydrogenase and thereby provides ammonia for the synthesis of carbamyl phosphate by carbamyl phosphate synthetase, the first step in the urea synthetic pathway. Alternatively glutamate may donate the amino group to aspartate via aspartate transaminase and thence condense with citrulline to form argininosuccinic acid.

The nitrogen-free analogs of essential amino acids might have at least two beneficial effects in urea cycle disorders. Because they serve as amino group acceptors in transamination reactions they could divert nonessential nitrogen away from urea synthesis and thus the requirement for urea synthesis could be reduced. A second possible benefit is

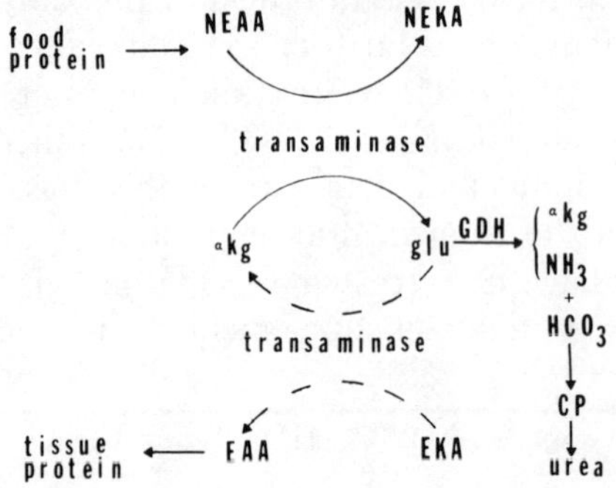

Figure 2. The dashed lines suggest a possible pathway whereby nitrogen may be diverted from urea synthesis to protein synthesis by the nitrogen-free analog of essential amino acids. Abbreviations: NEAA = nonessential amino acids, NEKA = nonessential keto acids, α-kg = alpha ketoglutarate, glu = glutamate, GDH = glutamate dehydrogenase, EKA = essential amino acid, CP = carbamyl phosphate.

the synthesis of essential amino acids, which may then be used for protein synthesis. In addition, certain keto acids, notably the branched-chain keto acids, have a regulatory effect on nitrogen sparing (1), the mechanism of which is unclear.

Are these analogs adequate nutritional substitutes for essential amino acids? They have been tested in animals and can with varying degrees of efficiency replace the corresponding essential amino acids in the diet (2). They have proven to be useful as nutritional supplements in the management of uremia in adults on protein-restricted diets (3). No adverse effects have been noted except occasional hypercalcemia (4). The use of sodium salts in nonuremic patients has prevented this side effect.

Can normal infants and children utilize these compounds? Figure 3 shows that when a mixture of keto acids is administered intravenously to an infant with ornithine transcarbamylase (OTC) deficiency there is a prompt increase in the plasma level of the corresponding amino acids. The left hand panel shows that at time zero "ketovaline," "ketoleucine," "ketoisoleucine," "ketomethionine," and phenylpyruvate were given intravenously. At the end of the infusion 4 hours later there was a dramatic increase of the corresponding amino acids, suggesting that prompt transamination of the keto acids occurred. Alloisoleucine (ALE) levels also increased because a racemic mixture of ketoisoleucine was given. The right hand panel shows a dramatic fall in the alanine level, suggesting that it was a nitrogen donor for transami-

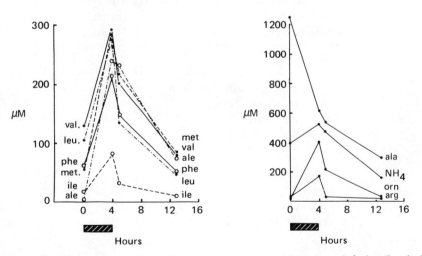

Figure 3. The plasma amino acid response to a 4-hour intravenous infusion (hatched area) of the ketone analogs of valine, leucine, isoleucine, methionine, and phenylalanine.

nation. The ornithine and arginine levels rose because arginine was included in the intravenous fluid.

Will these compounds promote growth in infants on marginal protein intakes? The nitrogen-free analogs were given to a normal newborn male infant who was thought to have ornithine transcarbamylase deficiency. Because he was the product of a woman who previously gave birth to an OTC-deficient male infant, his plasma ammonium level was followed carefully during the first 48 hours of life. The early hyperammonemia was erroneously interpreted as being diagnostic of OTC deficiency, and the child was treated as such. Beginning at 1 day of age, he was given a protein-restricted diet supplemented with a mixture of keto and hydroxy analogs of essential amino acids, plus the four remaining essential acids as such, plus arginine.

Table 1 shows the composition of the mixture of keto and hydroxy acids and amino acids he received in addition to a caloric intake of 120 cal/kg and pyridoxine. Note both the large amount of arginine and that three of the keto acids are given as the sodium salts. Figure 4 shows his protein intake, duration of ketoacid therapy, and weight gain. He was taking 120 Kcal/kg over this period of time. At 2 months of age an OTC assay was done on a liver biopsy and found to be within normal limits. The child had normal somatic and mental development while on keto acids despite a marginal protein intake. Evaluation at 1 year of age

Table 1   Composition of the Mixture Amino Acids and Their Nitrogen-Free Analogs Prescribed for Newborn Infants

Neonatal Mixture	Grams
"Ketoleucine", Na salt	1.15
S-"Ketoisoleucine" Na salt	0.84
"Ketovaline" Na salt	0.83
L-Phenyllactate, Ca salt	0.57
D,L-"Hydroxymethionine", Ca Salt	0.30
L-Lysine acetate	0.34
L-Histidine	0.23
L-Threonine	0.28
L-Tryptophan	0.15
L-Arginine	0.91
Total	5.60

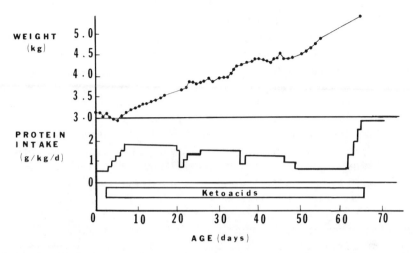

Figure 4. Clinical course of a normal infant whose intake was supplemented with a mixture of the nitrogen-free analogs of essential amino acids plus the remaining amino acids and arginine.

revealed his growth and neurological status to be normal with a score on the Cattell Infant Development Scale at a 12 to 14 month level. Based on the animal data and these studies in adults and infants it is apparent that keto acids are nontoxic nutritional substitutes for essential amino acids.

The 14 patients with urea cycle enzymopathies that we have studied are distributed as follows: three with carbamyl phosphate synthetase deficiency, seven with ornithine transcarbamylase deficiency, two with argininosuccinic acid synthetase deficiency, and one each with argininosuccinic acid lyase deficiency and arginase deficiency.

Figure 5 shows a diagram of the urea cycle demonstrating the metabolic consequences of a deficiency of carbamyl phosphate synthetase.

Carbamyl Phosphate Synthetase Deficiency

Gln
Ala → NH₄⁺ ⏸ CP → Cit — Asp
Glu   Pro ⇌ Orn   ASA
       Glu
              Arg
         Urea

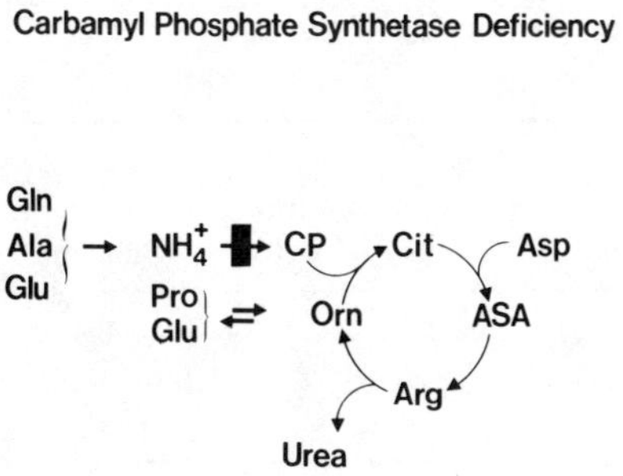

Figure 5. Metabolic consequences of carbamyl phosphate synthetase deficiency. The accumulated metabolites are Gln, Ala, Glu, NH₄⁺; the deficient metabolites are CP, Cit, Arg, and Urea; Pro, Orn, and Asp are unchanged, and the fate of ASA is unknown. Abbreviations: Gln = glutamine, Ala = alanine, Glu = glutamate, Pro = proline, CP = carbamyl phosphate, Cit = citrulline, Asp = aspartate, ASA = argininosuccinic acid, Arg = arginine.

The substrate immediately behind the block, ammonium, accumulates as do its precursors, glutamine, alanine, and glutamate. The substrates beyond the block decrease in concentration; there are low levels of carbamyl phosphate, citrulline, arginine, and urea. Ornithine levels are unchanged because ornithine may be synthesized from proline and glutamate. Aspartate levels are unchanged. The effect on argininosuccinic acid is unknown. It should be emphasized that in this defect and all others apart from arginase deficiency, the synthesis of arginine is impaired, thus making arginine an essential amino acid. Hence therapy for carbamyl phosphate synthetase deficiency should include arginine plus a mixture of analogs and essential amino acids designed to reduce the requirement for urea synthesis.

Table 2 shows the results of such therapy in patients with carbamyl phosphate synthetase deficiency. The infant was rescued from deep hyperammonemic coma by peritoneal dialysis, following which she was treated with the keto acid regimen. Throughout her 5 months of life her plasma ammonium level was within normal limits except for two episodes of hyperammonemic coma, the second of which caused her death. Although she appeared to be well during her first few weeks of life it became obvious by 3 months of age that she was severely brain damaged, perhaps as a result of her neonatal coma. The two older children with CPS deficiency responded to the regimen with normal plasma ammonium levels. One child, the first patient we reported (5), entered pubertal growth and demonstrated clinical improvement as shown by improved self help skills and accelerated growth. No clinical or biochemical change was noted in the other patient, although it was found that when a mixture of essential amino acids was substituted for keto acids she was less tolerant of protein as measured by the degree of hyperammonemia.

Figure 6 shows a diagram of the urea cycle demonstrating the metabolic consequences of a deficiency of ornithine transcarbamylase. The

Table 2   Response of Carbamyl Phosphate Synthetase Deficiency to Keto Acid Therapy

	Sex	Age at Onset of Therapy	Duration of Therapy	NH_4^+	Clinical Status During Therapy	Outcome
Neonates	F	7 days	5 months	WNL	Poor	Died
Children	F	13 years	3 years	WNL	Improved	Improved
	F	20 years	1 month	WNL	Unchanged	Unchanged

Ornithine Transcarbamylase Deficiency

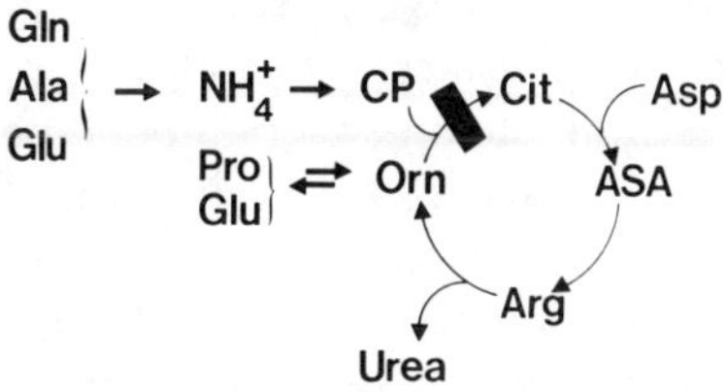

Figure 6. The metabolic consequences of ornithine transcarbamylase deficiency. The accumulated metabolites are Gln, Ala, Glu, NH_4^+, CP; the deficient metabolites are Cit, Arg, and Urea; Pro, Orn, and Asp are unchanged, and the fate of ASA is unknown. For abbreviations see Figure 5.

substrates (and their precursors) of the ornithine transcarbamylase reaction accumulate, whereas the products of the OTC reaction are decreased. The accumulated compounds include carbamyl phosphate, ammonium, glutamine, alanine, and glutamate. The deficient substrates include citrulline, arginine, and urea, Aspartate and ornithine are unchanged and the fate of argininosuccinic acid is unknown.

The metabolic consequences of this disease are virtually indistinguishable from those of carbamyl phosphate synthetase deficiency except that orotic aciduria is regularly observed (6), owing to the diversion of accumulated carbamyl phosphate into pyrimidine biosynthesis. We have therefore employed the same therapeutic regimen in this disorder as in carbamyl phosphate synthetase deficiency.

Table 3 summarizes the results of treatment of ornithine transcarbamylase deficiency in three male infants with the neonatal onset type, three older female children, and one male infant who was a variant of the usual X-linked disease. The clinical pattern exhibited by two of the male neonates in response to keto acid therapy is characteristic of our experience in treating the neonatal form of urea cycle enzymopathies. Two of these infants grew and developed normally, both had normal or near normal plasma levels of ammonium, and both died

Table 3   Response of Ornithine Transcarbamylase Deficiency to Keto Acid Therapy

	Sex	Age at Onset of Therapy	Duration of Therapy	NH_4^+	Clinical Status During Therapy	Outcome
Neonates	M	1d, 1d, 3d	2–6 months	WNL	Normal	2 died
Infants	M	8 mos	1.5 months	WNL	Normal	Died
Children	F	3y, 6y, 7y	6–7 months	WNL	1 improved, 2 unchanged	1 died

suddenly in hyperammonemic coma at 2 and 6 months of age. Although at the time of death no harbingers of impending hyperammonemic coma were recognized, in retrospect it was apparent that weeks before the 2-month-old infant died the plasma α-ketoglutarate level fell, followed in sequence by increases in plasma levels of glutamate and glutamine. One infant is currently alive although there is evidence of developmental delay after 7 months of therapy. His intake of the dietary supplement of analogs and essential amino acids is larger than that which we have employed in the other patients and in fact exceeds his protein intake by weight. The older male infant, presumably some sort of variant of X-linked disease, maintained a normal ammonium level during the short time he was on therapy, but died at 10 months of age in hyperammonemic coma. All three female children with partial OTC deficiency had normal or only slightly increased plasma ammonium levels in response to therapy, although little change was noted in their clinical course. Information on the fatal hyperammonemic episode of one of these children is still incomplete.

The pattern of precursor accumulation and product deficiencies in argininosuccinic acid synthetase deficiency is shown in Figure 7. Here, unlike carbamyl phosphate synthetase and ornithine transcarbamylase deficiency, there are large losses of the accumulated intermediate, citrulline, in the urine, which may constitute over 50% of total nitrogen excretion (7). Because citrulline contains one of the nitrogen atoms that ordinarily would be incorporated into urea, patients with argininosuccinic acid synthetase deficiency might be said to be citrullinotelic; they can excrete, at least in part, waste nitrogen as citrulline. In order to maintain this citrullinotelic state, however, there must be stoichiometric synthesis of ornithine either from dietary arginine or de novo from proline or glutamate via ornithine transaminase. Thus they have a substantially larger requirement for ornithine or arginine supplementation than children with defects of the first two enzymes of the cycle.

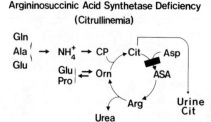

Argininosuccinic Acid Synthetase Deficiency
(Citrullinemia)

Figure 7. Metabolic consequences of argininosuccinic acid synthetase deficiency. The accumulated metabolites are Cit, Gln, Ala, Glu, NH_4^+, CP, and Urine Cit; the deficient metabolites are Urea, Arg, and ASA; Pro and Orn are unchanged. For abbreviations see Figure 5.

Table 4   Responses of AS Deficiency (Citrullinemia) to Keto Acid Therapy

	Sex	Age at Onset of Therapy	Duration of Therapy	NH$^+$	Clinical Status During Therapy	Outcome
Neonates	M	5 d, 20 d	7–8 months	WNL	Slight developmental delay	Died

Therefore therapy should include a large arginine supplement in addition to a mixture of analogs.

Table 4 summarizes the results of such treatment of two infants with the neonatal form of citrullinemia. In both cases plasma ammonium levels were maintained within normal limits and their somatic growth was within normal limits. These two patients demonstrated mild developmental delay with persistance of some primitive reflexes, perhaps as a result of their deep neonatal coma. However, both infants died within the first year of life in irreversible hyperammonemic coma, following a period of apparently excellent health. In one patient it was possible to establish his complete inability to excrete waste nitrogen as urea, both by postmortem enzymatic assay and by metabolic studies of the interdependence between arginine intake and urea excretion. The dietary arginine requirement to prevent hyperammonemia in this infant was found to be approximately 2.2 mmol/kg/day (7), a dose substantially larger than any other amino acid or analog. This dose was even larger, in fact, than would have been predicted on the basis of the loss of the ornithine skeleton of the arginine molecule as citrulline in the urine, suggesting that there was an excessive rate of diversion of arginine or ornithine into other pathways.

Figure 8 shows the effects of a deficiency of argininosuccinic acid

Argininosuccinic Acid Lyase Deficiency
(Argininosuccinic Aciduria)

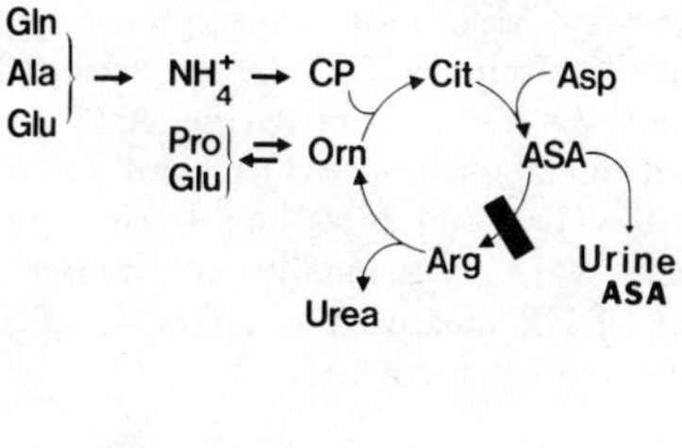

Figure 8. Metabolic consequences of argininosuccinic acid lyase deficiency. The accumulated metabolites are Gln, Ala, Glu, Cit, ASA, Asp, and Urine ASA; the deficient metabolites are Orn, Arg and Urea; NH$_4^+$ and Pro are unchanged, and the fate of CP is unknown. For abbreviations see Figure 5.

lyase on the substrates and products of the urea cycle. Virtually all the substrates behind the block accumulate, although ammonium may be normal even when there is accumulation of other labile nitrogenous substances (9). We have no explanation for this apparent paradox. Another finding that is in contrast to the previously described defects is the low ornithine level. We would like to suggest that disposal of waste nitrogen in argininosuccinic acid lyase deficiency may not be impaired. Both nitrogen atoms which ultimately are excreted as urea are present in argininosuccinic acid, which itself is rapidly excreted in the urine. In order to maintain this high excretion, argininosuccinic acid must be synthesized from ornithine. Thus, the rapid loss of ornithine skeletons as argininosuccinic acid might account for the low levels of ornithine. An appropriate intake of protein and arginine should restore patients with argininosuccinic acid lyase deficiency to normal. Although high levels of plasma argininosuccinic acid may be toxic, recent data suggest that they may not be (8). Sufficient arginine intake not only would prevent arginine deficiency but also could supply ornithine skeletons required for argininosuccinic excretion. Additional ornithine for this purpose may be synthesized via ornithine transaminase. The delta amino nitrogen of such de novo synthesized ornithine would represent a third atom of nitrogen to be excreted as waste nitrogen in argininosuccinic acid. It is not clear that these patients would benefit from nitrogen-free analogs because there is no defect in waste nitrogen excretion.

Only one patient with AL deficiency was treated with keto acids. Her clinical state was unchanged after therapy.

Figure 9 shows the urea cycle as it is affected by a deficiency of arginase. This is the only one of these diseases in which arginine is not an essential amino acid. In contrast to all other urea cycle defects only the substrate immediately behind the block accumulates. Hyperammonemia is only an occasional finding. Ornithine levels are probably low because its synthesis fails to keep pace with its loss as arginine in the urine. The progressive neurological deterioration that occurs in

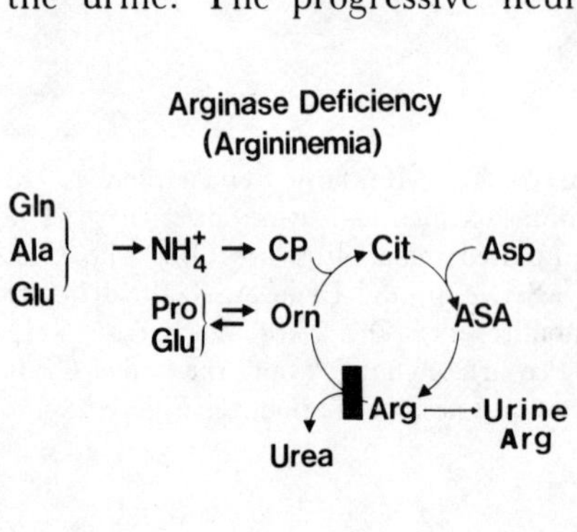

Arginase Deficiency (Argininemia)

Figure 9. Metabolic consequences of arginase deficiency. The accumulated metabolites are Arg and Urine Arg; the deficient metabolites are Orn and Urea; Gln, Ala, Glu, and NH_4^+ are unchanged, although NH_4^+ occasionally accumulates; the fate of CP and ASA is unknown. For abbreviations see Figure 5.

these patients is probably related to the high levels of arginine and its metabolic products rather than to hyperammonemia. The single arginase-deficient patient we have treated with keto acids was unchanged after therapy, as one would predict. Clearly an arginine-restricted diet should be helpful. Snyderman has reported beneficial results in treating such patients with an arginine-restricted diet supplemented with essential amino acids (10).

SUMMARY

Our experience with nitrogen-free analog therapy of these disorders indicates that these compounds are adequate nutritional supplements which are non-toxic and which promote mental and somatic growth. They prevent or reduce hyperammonemia for varying periods of time in three of these disorders, but as yet have not prevented hyperammonemic coma and death in infants with complete enzyme deficiencies. Further work will be necessary to determine how impending hyperammonemic coma can be detected before it becomes irreversible, as well as to improve the therapy of hyperammonemic coma when it develops.

REFERENCES

1.   D. G. Sapir, E. O. Owen, T. Pozefsky, et. al., *J. Clin. Invest.*, **54**, 974 (1974).
2.   K. W. Chow and M. Walser, *J. Nutr.*, **104**, 1208 (1974).
3.   M. Walser, A. W. Coulter, S. Dighe, et. al., *J. Clin. Invest.*, **52**, 678 (1973).
4.   W. E. Mitch, B. Gelman, and M. Walser, 10th Annual Meeting of the American Society of Nephrology, p. 78A, (1977).
5.   M. Batshaw, S. Brusilow, and M. Walser, *New Engl. J. Med.*, **292**, 1085 (1975).
6.   B. Levin, V. G. Oberholzer, and L. Sinclair, *Lancet*, **2**, 170 (1969).
7.   M. Walser, M. Batshaw, G. Sherwood, B. Robinson, and S. Brusilow, *Clin. Sci. and Molecular Med.*, **53**, 173 (1977).
8.   A. G. F. Davidson, et al., *Clin. Res.*, **24**, 186A (1976).
9.   S. Brusilow, M. Walser, and M. Batshaw, Unpublished observations.
10.   S. E. Snyderman, C. Sansaricq, W. J. Chen, P. M. Norton, and J. V. Phansalkar, *J. Ped.*, **90**, 563 (1977).

PART 3

Carbohydrates

5

Lactose Intolerance

THEODORE M. BAYLESS, M.D.

Associate Professor of Medicine, Johns Hopkins University School of Medicine, Johns Hopkins Hospital, Baltimore, Maryland

and

DAVID M. PAIGE, M.D., M.P.H.

Associate Professor of Maternal and Child Health, Johns Hopkins University School of Hygiene and Public Health, Johns Hopkins Hospital, Baltimore, Maryland

In this chapter we shall discuss first the digestion of milk sugar lactose and how disorders of lactose digestion and absorption result in potential milk intolerance. Our second subject will be a classification of cases of lactose intolerance. Third, we shall discuss the significance of a person's being lactose intolerant. Most lactose tolerance testing is performed with large amounts of sugar equivalent to one or two quarts of milk. What does it mean if a person cannot digest that much milk? Fourth, we will concentrate on the management of the individual patient who is recognized to be milk intolerant. Last, and perhaps of most importance to this audience, we will discuss the controversies concerning the significance of lactose intolerance in nutritional planning for populations. Should milk be included in food programs for all ages regardless of genetic background and tendency toward milk intolerance?

DISACCHARIDE DIGESTION

Ordinarily the disaccharides such as the milk sugar lactose are digested by very specific enzymes in the brush border lining of the intestinal mucosa (Fig. 1). There is a specific lactase which splits lactose to the simple sugars, glucose and galactose, which are absorbed. Lactose itself

79

cannot be absorbed without digestion. Similarly, there is an enzyme for digesting sucrose and disorders in the activity of this enzyme, sucrase, will be discussed in Chapter 6. Although there are at least three maltases, clinical defects in maltose digestion have not been identified.

When an individual with normal intestinal lactase levels drinks the lactose equivalent to one or two quarts of milk the lactase is able to digest the lactose to simple sugars which are easily absorbed, with a resultant rise in the blood glucose level, usually over 20 or 25 mg/dl. The subject remains asymptomatic. The situation differs in a person with low or inadequate lactase levels, a condition sometimes referred to as lactase deficiency. The undigested lactose remains in the intestine and acts as an osmotic load, drawing fluid and electrolytes into the intestine. Next, as the undigested sugar enters the colon, it is fermented by bacteria, forming short-chain acids which are even more osmotically active. In addition, the bowel contents become quite acidic. These conditions interfere with the absorption of fluids and electrolytes in the colon, with diarrhea as the result in some individuals. There is also fermentation of the undigested sugar to hydrogen and carbon dioxide, so that flatulence and gaseous distention are very common symptoms in lactose intolerant people who drink 1 or 2 glasses of milk. One can test a subject's ability

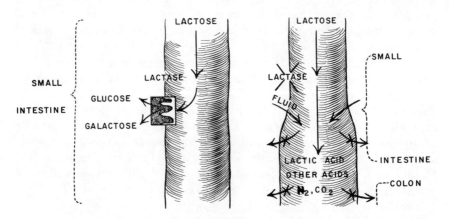

Figure 1. When lactase levels are normal, as on the left, lactose is hydrolyzed in the small intestine into absorbable glucose and galactose. There is a rise in blood sugar and no symptoms are produced. With low lactase levels, as on the right, the disaccharide's continued presence causes fluid flow into the gut and interferes with fluid reabsorption in the small intestine and colon. The undigested sugar is fermented to short-chain acids with acidification of bowel contents and production of gases. All these events combine to produce bloating, flatulence, and in some instances diarrhea.

to digest lactose by giving a tolerance test load to determine if any symptoms are produced and if the blood glucose rises normally. Pediatricians make use of the fact that acids are formed in the colon by measuring the pH in the stool to detect the presence of lactose intolerance. One can also measure the amount or the concentration of hydrogen in breath, since this gives some measure of the amount of undigested sugar that reaches the colon and is fermented. The actual level of lactase activity can be measured directly in intestinal biopsy specimens.

DEFINITIONS

The terms *low lactase levels* and *lactase deficiency* can be used interchangeably. I prefer the term low lactase levels because, as we shall discuss later, this may be the normal situation in man. *Lactose intolerance* means that a person cannot digest a large lactose load equivalent to one or two quarts of milk as shown by a flat blood sugar rise of less than 20 or 25 mg/dl. Such people are usually symptomatic, noticing gas, bloating, or even a laxative effect. *Lactose malabsorption* means that a subject has an inadequate rise in blood sugar but no symptoms are reported. *Lactose tolerance* applies to a person who can take the equivalent of one or two quarts of milk with no symptoms and a normal rise in blood sugar. *Milk intolerance,* by our current understanding, refers to a person who, after ingesting some quantity of milk, gets symptoms—usually mild bloating, gas, or cramps. Some people who have low lactase levels will be asymptomatic with one glass of skim milk, whereas others will have to drink two or three glasses of milk before symptoms are noted. There are some patients who are symptomatic with even a quarter glass of milk. Hence at present this definition of milk intolerance is not really absolute. In the future the term may also be used to refer to subjects in whom evidence of maldigestion of the contents of a glass of milk can be demonstrated.

CLASSIFICATION OF LACTOSE MALDIGESTION

Relatively low lactase levels apparently occur in the low birth weight or premature infant for the first 1 or 2 weeks of life. The clinical significance of this relative lactase deficiency in premature infants has not been clearly established. *Congenital lactase deficiency,* which is very rare, is a recessively inherited trait. Recognition at birth is essential because if it is not recognized and the infant is fed milk, diarrhea and malnutrition ensue with resultant mucosal damage, which leads to secondary disaccharidase deficiency and carbohydrate malabsorption, finally resulting in more severe malnutrition. If this vicious cycle continues, the infant may die of malnutrition. This is a very rare congenital defect. *Secondary lactase deficiency,* subsequent to damage of the gut, such as in the infant with infectious gastroenteritis, is much more common. If the intestine is damaged severely, levels of all of the disaccharidases, sucrase, maltase, and lactase, are decreased. Lactase is the most easily damaged and its recovery is the most prolonged. A *postweaning decrease in lactase levels* is a common occurrence. Subjects acquire low lactase levels after infancy, perhaps at age 3 or 4 years, or during early teenage (1). It is generally agreed that these low lactase levels are under genetic control as an autosomal recessive trait. The major portion of this discussion will deal with these individuals. There are also patients who can not tolerate moderate amounts of lactose even though they have normal lactase levels. As an example, a patient who has had gastric surgery for peptic ulcer may not be able to digest milk feedings. This condition may also occur with patients given large amounts of milk as a tube feeding which is rapidly delivered to the intestine. Even though these individuals have normal lactase levels, they cannot digest the large lactose load quickly, and thus become symptomatic.

PREVALENCE OF LOW LACTASE LEVELS

Dr. Rosensweig and I studied the prevalence of low lactase levels in 20 healthy black and 20 healthy white adults and found that among the blacks 14, or 70%, had low lactase levels as compared to only 1 of the whites. The difference between these groups led us to suggest that lactase levels were under genetic control (2).

Dr. Shi Shung Huang and I subsequently studied Oriental adults. Of 20 Oriental house officers, nurses, and dieticians, 19 had symptoms with a lactose load and were lactose intolerant. This led us to believe that lactose intolerance was extremely common in many populations and we suggested that the bulk of the world's population probably had low lactase levels (3).

Some of the current information on the prevalence of low lactase levels or lactose intolerance is listed in Table 1. The prevalence is less

Table 1   Generalizations on Prevalence of Lactose Intolerance in Adults

<15%	60–80%	>80%
Scandinavians	Mexican Americans	Formosans
Northwestern Europeans	U.S. Indians[b]	Japanese
White Australians	U.S. Jews	South Nigerians
White Americans[a]	U.S. Blacks	Bantu[b]
Batulsi, Fulani		Eskimos[b]

[a] Of Scandinavian or Western European extraction.
[b] Tribal differences in prevalence.

than 15% in white Americans whose ancestors were from Scandinavia or northwestern Europe. There are some very interesting tribes in Africa who have a long history of dairying and who apparently have adequate lactase levels. Their dairying history dates back before A.D. 1500. There is a 60 to 80% prevalence of lactose intolerance among Mexican American adults, and United States Indians, Jews, and blacks. The prevalence is even higher in some Oriental, Bantu, African, and some United States Indian and some Eskimo tribes.

GENETIC CONTROL OF LACTASE ACTIVITY

What is the reason for this worldwide high prevalence? Is it an adaptation to decreased milk intake? We do not think so. Feeding milk does not reverse this, and conversely abstaining from milk does not lower lactase levels. We do not think that it is due to intestinal damage. Most workers agree that it is an inherited trait with a delayed clinical expression. The enzyme is present in adequate amounts at birth, and then for some undetermined reason decreases during childhood. There is a pattern of a falling level of lactase after weaning in almost every animal species that has been studied. This was not thought to be true in man, since all of us have been encouraged to drink milk throughout our adult life, but our work and that of others indicates that a pattern of a postweaning falloff in lactase probably does occur in most of the world's populations. The rate of fall in lactase activity varies.

In Mestizo in Peru, Dr. Paige and his colleagues found that by the age of 3 to 5 years, most of the subjects were already lactose intolerant (4). Other groups with a similarly rapid postweaning decrease in lactase activity include Pima Indians in Arizona (5), Baganda in Uganda (6), and Yoruba in Nigeria (7). These last are believed to be ancestors of many of the United States blacks.

An autosomal recessive inheritance has been hypothesized. There are some supporting data from Indian tribes in Minnesota and from Arizona. If both parents were normal, it was expected that 25% of the offspring would be lactose intolerant, and a Mayo Clinic group observed that 40% were. If one parent was lactase deficient, 50% of the offspring were predicted to be deficient, and they observed 65%. If both parents were lactose intolerant, 93% of their children were found to be lactose intolerant (8). There have been a number of other family studies which confirm that this probably is a recessive trait (5,7,9).

Measurement of actual lactase levels in a mixed population of adults demonstrated that unaffected blacks, that is, those with "normal" lactase levels, had a mean enzyme level about half that of unaffected whites, suggesting that most of the blacks were heterozygotes, while the white population contained both heterozygotes and homozygotes for adequate lactase levels. Our studies supported the concept that low lactase levels are a non-sex-linked autosomal recessive trait (10).

Lactase is not an inducible enzyme; that is, feeding lactose will not increase levels and abstaining does not lower levels in an individual subject. Despite this lack of enzyme adaptation in the individual there is some very interesting work by Dr. Frederick Simoons and others suggesting that the milk drinking habits of a person's ancient ancestors play a role in one's capacity to digest lactose.

If your ancestors were dairying and milk consuming people prior to A.D. 1500 you probably have adequate lactase activity. It is their thought that it is normal not to have high lactase levels as an adult and that this enzyme adapted to the needs of milk drinkers before A.D. 1500 (11).

Utilizing current prevalence data, we would estimate that there are approximately 30 million lactose intolerant people in the United States. Those people would be bothered by the equivalent of two quarts of milk. What does that mean? Are these 30 million "potentially" milk intolerant? This is where the controversies arise. We shall discuss various views on this question.

CONSEQUENCES OF LACTOSE INTOLERANCE

What are the consequences of having low lactase levels? There are some people who are drinking milk and are experiencing overt symptoms.

Patients with irritable bowel syndrome or postgastrectomy diarrhea may not have recognized the relationship of their symptoms to milk ingestion. These patients, who are milk intolerant, may be symptomatic after drinking one or two glasses of milk at a time. The gas, cramps, or distension start 2 to 3 hours later. In some subjects the relationship of milk to symptoms is not as obvious. This has been true for abdominal pain in school-age children who have not recognized the relationship of the pain to milk.

EVALUATION OF POSSIBLE MILK INTOLERANCE

Suspecting the diagnosis is probably the key point. The patients can be asked to discontinue or lessen their milk and ice cream intake for a few days to see if symptoms remit. They then might test themselves with several glasses of milk at home to see if they again become symptomatic. A lactose tolerance test could be employed if needed to confirm the diagnosis. Breath hydrogen analysis will probably be more available in the future.

MANAGEMENT OF MILK INTOLERANCE

The main form of treatment is to decrease the amount of milk and milk products that the patient consumes to an amount that does not cause symptoms (12,13). The milk intolerant patient does not have to avoid all milk intake, only to limit his intake to tolerable amounts. Dr. Jack Welsh of Oklahoma has surveyed a series of hospitals in this country and has found that many hospitals do not have a low lactose diet or a lactose-restricted diet in their formulary. Some use the galactose-free diet for galactosemics, which is entirely free of lactose. This is too strict a diet for this problem.

It is our impression that giving milk with a meal will lessen symptoms. Dr. Marshall Bedine and I reported that feeding lactose with a meal would double the threshold for symptom production (14). This has not been a universal finding. A recent paper by Jones, Latham, and their co-workers reported that giving lactose with meals did not lessen symptoms (15). We do hear anecdotes of people with lactose intolerance who are able to tolerate more milk if they take it with a meal. We assume that the meal delays gastric emptying and dilutes the lactose load. Lactose hydrolized milk is one alternative if one does wish to use a dairy product in the lactose intolerant person.

CLINICAL SETTINGS FOR MILK INTOLERANCE

Milk intolerance should be suspected in patients from population groups with a high prevalence of lactose intolerance or in someone who has a family history of milk intolerance. One should at least consider the possibility of milk intolerance as a diagnosis if a person with gastrointestinal symptoms is consuming one or two glasses of milk at a time. Increased milk consumption, as for peptic ulcer or for pregnancy, is a setting for the appearance of the clinical symptoms of lactose intolerance. Current nutritional brochures recommend that pregnant women consume three 8-ounce cups of milk each day for the first 3 months, and four cups thereafter. We believe that some lactose intolerant individuals would become symptomatic with that increased intake. Some nutritional supplements, including many of the common tube feedings, contain lactose, so that the nutritionist must be aware of potential lactose or milk induced symptoms when working with patients who might be lactose intolerant. The beneficial effects of recognizing milk intolerance can be seen in patients with irritable bowel syndrome. Often their symptoms can be alleviated simply by limiting the amount of milk ingested.

CLINICAL CONSEQUENCES OF LACTOSE INTOLERANCE

What amounts of milk should we be recommending for use in feeding programs? Should lactose intolerance be considered when one recommends three or four glasses of milk per day for people? There is controversy over this issue. The *Dairy Council Digest* in May/June 1977 suggests that people are using false logic or are believing myths about milk and therefore are not consuming particular dairy products, thus depriving themselves of this contribution to their nutrition. Studies have been produced supporting many different opinions on the clinical significance of lactose intolerance.

It is generally accepted that low lactase levels are prevalent and genetically controlled. What is still controversial is the relationship of lactose intolerance to milk intolerance. Are any of the people who are lactose intolerant also milk intolerant? Are half of them milk intolerant? A quarter? A tenth? What is the percentage? Is there any effect of lactose intolerance on milk consumption? Do people who are milk intolerant and have recognized this fact drink less milk? Is there any problem with the absorption of the nutrients from a glass of milk? If a person cannot digest the lactose is he then absorbing the other water-soluble nutrients in a glass of milk? And finally, what recommendations should be offered in reference to food programs? (16).

AWARENESS OF MILK INTOLERANCE

In terms of awareness of milk intolerance, about two-thirds of a series of randomly selected adults who are lactose intolerant and who are in communities where milk is being consumed will realize that milk causes gas, or at times acts as a laxative for them. This is not a specific symptom because approximately one-third of lactose tolerant adults will give such a history (17).

MILK INDUCED SYMPTOMS

Another measure of the clinical significance of lactose intolerance would be to determine what percentage of such subjects becomes symptomatic after drinking usually consumed amounts of milk. In a selected population of 20 milk intolerant adults with low lactase levels 75% became symptomatic when they drank 12 g of lactose, equivalent to one glass of milk. Two had symptoms with the lactose in one-quarter of a glass of milk. None had symptoms with equal amounts of sucrose or glucose and galactose. The amount of lactose in one-half glass of milk will produce fluid accumulation in the intestine (18) and will cause a rise in breath hydrogen in some people. A recent study from Scandinavia presents similar data and confirms our observations (19). Further studies in an unselected population gave similar results. Forty-four randomly selected lactose intolerant adults were given a glass of low fat milk without other food and 59% had symptoms. The main symptoms noted were gas, distention, and cramps. These adults rarely noted diarrhea after drinking milk.

Based on these investigations we estimate that half of lactose intolerant adults will have symptoms with one glass of milk taken fasting. This estimate is not universally accepted. Other workers have found that the threshold for "significant symptoms" is somewhat higher. Stephenson and Latham reported that only 7% of volunteer subjects had mild symptoms with 15 g of lactose (20). If you calculate their data differently and combine figures for one glass of milk and two glasses of milk, 65 to 81% had symptoms with two glasses of milk. Hence they found a somewhat higher threshold for symptoms with milk than we reported. Other studies on the tolerance of milk which differ from ours have used lactose or milk taken with food, and it is our thought that this will raise the threshold for symptoms and perhaps lessen their severity (21).

Results in teenagers and children have also been somewhat at variance. Mitchell and co-workers reported that 6 of 13 lactose intolerant teenagers had symptoms with one glass of milk. Unfortunately, some of the other studies in children have been done by feeding milk with peanut butter sandwiches or with a meal, and they have found a higher threshold (21,22). A recent study in American Indian teenagers and adults reported an average threshold of 30 g, in contrast to our reports of a threshold of about 12 g in about half the lactose intolerant subjects.

MILK CONSUMPTION

How do these findings affect the consumption of milk? Are people's milk drinking habits influenced by their lactose digesting ability? When one compares beverage consumption in the United States between 1960 and 1973, there has been a 22% decrease in milk consumption and, unfortunately, a 111% increase in soft drink consumption. Does lactose play any role in the decreased milk drinking? We do not know.

It is well known to nutritionists that a number of factors influence any food consumption, and milk is no exception. Income, family size and composition, the attitude of the family toward milk, knowledge, attitudes, and practices are all important variables that will influence milk consumption. We believe that lactose intolerance is an additional factor, but again, not everyone agrees. It is important at least to consider whether lactose intolerance plays any role, since milk is so important in many feeding programs. For example, the United States Department of Agriculture, in fiscal year 1976, dispensed 7175 billion one-half pints of milk to school children. One can determine milk consumption by taking the carton off the tray after a meal and measuring the milk left in it. If the subject consumed only one-quarter of the carton or less, then we considered him a nondrinker. Among lactose intolerant adults, 30% of one series were nondrinkers compared to 10% of the lactose tolerant patients. Thus about one-third of the lactose intolerant patients were not drinking the milk that was given on their tray (17). Our original studies on milk drinking were in elementary school pupils. Dr. David Paige and his colleagues measured the actual milk consumption and found that 20% of over 300 young black children drank less than half of the milk with their hot meal, as compared to about 10% of approximately 200 whites.

Lactose tolerance tests indicated that lactose intolerance was very common among a sample of the black milk nondrinkers, suggesting that there was some correlation between abnormal lactose tolerance tests and not drinking milk (23). A recent study by Stephenson, Latham, and Jones debates this finding. They reported that 10% of both whites and blacks, with no racial difference, did not drink milk. They did not do tolerance tests. Their data do, however, show that black females were consuming less milk than any other group. However in their conclusions they challenge our thought that milk consumption is affected by lactose intolerance (24). A partial explanation for the differences may be based on age differences. Dr. Paige and his colleagues did not observe significant milk rejection before the age of 8 years. If our data are divided into those less than 5, 5 to 7, and over 8, there is a 22% milk rejection rate among those children subjects over age 8, but below 8 there was not as clear a pattern. It is our preliminary thought that age 8 might be the point after which one must be concerned about milk consumption related to lactose intolerance in populations with a high prevalence of lactose intolerance.

ABSORPTION OF NUTRIENTS IN MILK

There are some reasons to believe that lactose intolerant subjects may not absorb all of the nutrients in a glass of milk. Lactose absorption from a glass of milk as reflected in blood sugar rise is less in lactose intolerant teenagers than in lactose tolerant controls. This difference can be corrected by the use of lactose hydrolyzed milk. Evidence indicates that there is decreased absorption of at least the carbohydrate portion of a glass of milk in some lactose intolerant subjects.

FEEDING PROGRAM CONSIDERATIONS

We believe that those planning feeding programs in populations with a high prevalence of lactose intolerance should be aware of the possibility of milk-induced symptoms. We think that actual consumption should be evaluated as well as questions about symptoms. Fermented or hydrolyzed milk products could be considered if milk rejection is observed or its symptoms are occurring. Other protein or calcium sources could be considered for populations, especially for subjects over age 8, in whom lactose intolerance may be a problem. One should clearly be alert to potential milk intolerance in teenagers and in adults in high prevalence populations (25).

REFERENCES

1. D. H. Alpers and B. Seetharam, *N. Engl. J. Med.*, **296**, 1047 (1977).
2. T. M. Bayless and N. S. Rosensweig, *J.A.M.A.*, **197**, 968 (1966).
3. S. S. Huang and T. M. Bayless, *N. Engl. J. Med.*, **276**, 283 (1967).
4. D. M. Paige, E. Leonardo, A. Cordano, T. B. Adrianzen, J. Nakashima, and G. G. Graham, *Am. J. Clin. Nutr.* **25**, 297 (1972).
5. J. D. Johnson, F. J. Simoons, R. Hurwitz, A. Grang, et al., *Gastroenterology*, **73**, 1299 (1977).
6. G. C. Cook, *Brit. Med. J.*, **1**, 527 (1967).
7. O. Ransome-Kuti, N. Kretchmer, J. D. Johnson, et al., *Gastroenterology*, **68**, 431 (1975).
8. A. D. Newcomer, P. J. Thomas, D. B. McGill, et al., *Gastroenterology*, **72**, 234 (1977).
9. T. Sahi, M. Isokoski, J. Jussila, et al., *Lancet*, **2**, 823 (1973).
10. T. M. Bayless, N. L. Christopher, and S. H. Boyer, *J. Clin. Invest.*, **48**, 6a (1969).
11. F. J. Simoons, *Am. J. Digest. Dis.*, **18**, 595 (1973).
12. M. S. Hardinge, J. B. Swarner, and H. Crooks, *J. Am. Diet. Assn.*, **46**, 197 (1965).
13. D. Lee and C. Lillibridge, *Am. J. Clin. Nutr.*, **29**, 428 (1976).
14. M. S. Bedine and T. M. Bayless, *Clin. Res.*, **20**, 448 (1972).
15. D. V. Jones and M. C. Latham, *J. Trop. Pediatr.*, **20**, 262 (1974).
16. D. M. Paige, et al., *Am. J. Clin. Nutr.*, **28**, 818 (1975).
17. T. M. Bayless, B. Rothfeld, C. Massa, L. Wise, D. Paige, and M. S. Bedine, *N. Engl. J. Med.*, **292**, 1156 (1975).
18. M. S. Bedine and T. M. Bayless, *Gastroenterology*, **65**, 735 (1973).
19. E. Gudmand-Hoyer and K. Simoney, *Digest. Dis.*, **22**, 177 (1977).
20. L. S. Stephenson and M. C. Latham, *Am. J. Clin. Nutr.*, **27**, 296 (1974).
21. A. D. Newcomer, D. B. McGill, P. J. Thomas, and A. F. Hofmann, *Gastroenterology*, **74**, 44 (1978).
22. C. Garza and N. S. Scrimshaw, *Am. J. Clin. Nutr.*, **29**, 192, (1976).
23. D. M. Paige, T. M. Bayless, G. D. Ferry, and G. G. Graham, *Johns Hopkins Med. J.*, **129**, 163 (1971).
24. L. S. Stephenson, M. C. Latham, and D. V. Jones, *J. Amer. Dietetic Assn.*, **71**, 248 (1977).
25. F. J. Simoons, J. D. Johnson, and N. Kretchmer, *Pediatrics*, **50**, 98 (1977).

6

Other Carbohydrate Intolerances

NORTON S. ROSENSWEIG, M.D.

Division of Gastroenterology and Nutrition, Department of Medicine, North Shore
University Hospital, Manhasset, New York; and Cornell University Medical College,
New York, New York

Chapter 5 by Dr. Bayless deals exclusively with milk and lactose intolerance due to lactase deficiency. This chapter is devoted primarily to the effect of dietary sugars on intestinal enzymes and to selected other carbohydrate intolerances. Most of these latter conditions are very uncommon to downright rare compared with lactase deficiency.

LACTOSE FEEDING AND LACTASE DEFICIENCY

Although the current treatment of milk and lactose intolerance is based on lactose restriction, some early studies focused on treating the lactase deficiency by attempted induction of the enzyme with milk or lactose feeding (1–3). Cuatrecasas et al. felt that human lactase activity might be inducible but were unable to increase lactase activity in deficient patients by prolonged milk feeding (1). Although symptoms of milk intolerance decreased markedly after a week or so of feeding, enzyme activity did not increase. Even when a quart of milk or more was fed daily to lactase deficient patients for up to one year, no increase in lactase activity could be demonstrated (2,3).

In studies with normal volunteer subjects, lactase activity was unchanged despite feeding of up to 450 g of lactose daily (4). In reciprocal studies, complete removal of lactose from the diet for as long as 2 months in normal subjects or for many years in galactosemic patients failed to alter lactase activity in the normals or show any increased incidence of lactose intolerance in the galactosemics (5–7). Therefore, current evidence suggests that human lactase activity is under genetic control. I have reviewed the topic of dietary or genetic control of lactase activity in man in depth elsewhere (8).

DISACCHARIDASE ADAPTATION

Although human lactase activity does not adapt to milk or lactose feeding, the activity of other disaccharidases adapts readily to certain dietary sugars (9,10). Specifically, sucrose feeding, as compared to equicaloric glucose feeding, significantly increases sucrase and maltase activities but does not alter lactase activity (9). This response occurs in 2 to 5 days and is similar to the renewal time of the small intestine (10). Therefore, the sucrose effect acts initially through the crypt cell and manifests itself by intestinal cell migration up the villus and maturation of the epithelial cell (10).

When maltose, lactose, or galactose feeding was compared to glucose, there was no change in sucrase and maltase activities. However, when fructose, the end product of sucrose hydrolysis, was fed, there was an increase in sucrase and maltase activities identical to that obtained with sucrose feeding. This suggests that fructose is the active principle in the sucrose molecule and also demonstrates that specific substrate is not required for an adaptive response. Actually, a gradient of responses is seen since feeding glucose increases sucrase and maltase activities above those seen with a carobhydrate-free diet but still significantly less than feeding sucrose or fructose (11).

The fact that fructose, a monosaccharide, could increase sucrase activity and also be absorbed without prior disaccharidase hydrolysis, suggested that fructose might be used to treat sucrase deficiency. This hypothesis was soon tested by Greene et al., who fed fructose to a 7-year-old girl with sucrase-isomaltase deficiency (12). She had a long history of chronic diarrhea and failure to gain weight. Extensive original work-up was negative with normal jejunal histology, but disaccharidase assay revealed low sucrase and isomaltase activities. With fructose feeding, sucrase activity increased fourfold (but was still below normal), the isomaltase doubled, and the sucrose tolerance test improved significantly. When treated with a sucrose-restricted, 20% fructose diet, she gained weight, became asymptomatic, and was able to tolerate modest amounts of sucrose. Although significant success was achieved with this patient, it is necessary to treat many more patients in this manner before any general conclusions may be drawn.

OTHER CARBOHYDRATE INTOLERANCES

Although the above data suggest that fructose in the diet may be useful in treating sucrase-isomaltase deficiency, there are rare metabolic disorders in which normal fructose metabolism is blocked. Essential fructosuria is a benign condition without symptoms in which fructose is found in the urine, usually on routine urine screening tests (13). It is due to a defect in hepatic fructokinase (probably small intestine as well), which is the first enzyme in the fructose metabolic pathway:

$$\text{fructose} \xrightarrow{\text{fructokinase}} \text{fructose-1-phosphate}$$

In this harmless condition, fructose is present in the urine only after fructose ingestion. Fructose is absorbed normally from the small intestine but is not metabolized in the liver. Accordingly, blood fructose will rise to high levels (above 25 mg per 100 ml) during oral fructose tolerance tests. The patient remains asymptomatic and glucose and galactose metabolism are normal. It is inherited as an autosomal recessive trait.

Hereditary fructose intolerance is a much more serious condition with significant symptoms from fructose ingestion (13). It is due to a defect of the activity of fructose-1-phosphate aldolase, the second enzyme in the fructose metabolic pathway.

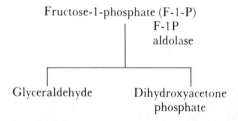

Unlike the case with essential fructosuria, here the ingestion of fructose leads to vomiting, hypoglycemia, and hypophosphatemia. Chronic fructose ingestion in children leads to failure to thrive, vomiting, jaundice, hepatomegaly, splenomegaly, hyperbilirubinemia, albuminuria, and aminoaciduria and possibly death if untreated. Older children usually develop a marked aversion for sweets and fruits. The administration of fructose leads to fructosemia, fructosuria, hypoglycemia, and hypophosphatemia.

The condition is a hereditary disorder consistent with an autosomal recessive trait. The standard treatment is to restrict the ingestion of all foods containing fructose. The other monosaccharides, glucose and galactose, are absorbed and metabolized normally and are completely satisfactory carbohydrate sources. When it was shown that oral folic acid could increase human jejunal glycolytic enzyme activities (14) Greene et al. used high doses of folate to treat a patient with this disorder (15). Further studies are needed before any definite conclusions can be drawn.

GALACTOSEMIA

Classic galactosemia is a rare disorder characterized by an inability to metabolize galactose in a normal fashion (16). It is due to a deficiency of the enzyme galactose-1-phosphate uridyl transferase.

$$\text{Galactose-1-phosphate} + \text{UDP-glucose} \xrightarrow{\text{transferase}}$$
$$\text{UDP-galactose} + \text{glucose-1-phosphate}$$

It is inherited as an autosomal recessive trait and occurs in approximately 1 in 50,000 to 100,000 births. The symptoms usually begin days to several weeks after birth and consist of vomiting, poor nutrition, failure to thrive, jaundice, hepatomegaly, and then evidence of liver disease. Cataracts and mental retardation occur later on.

The enzymatic defect leads to the accumulation of galactose-1-phosphate and galactose in the tissues and galactitol in the lens. This leads to the cataracts. The diagnosis is made by demonstration of the enzyme deficiency in red blood cells. Treatment centers around removal of all foods containing galactose from the diet. If treatment is instituted promptly, there is rapid improvement in the patient; and if it is begun early enough, mental retardation can be avoided.

A second type of galactosemia called galactokinase deficiency galactosemia has been described recently. This is an autosomal recessive condition characterized only by cataract formation. Treatment is a low galactose diet.

GLUCOSE-GALACTOSE MALABSORPTION

Glucose-galactose malabsorption is an extremely rare hereditary disorder characterized by severe watery diarrhea essentially from birth (17). Its mode of inheritance is autosomal recessive. Carbohydrates found in the stool are primarily monosaccharide. There is normal small intestinal, mucosal histology and disaccharidase activity. Disaccharides are hydrolyzed normally, but glucose and galactose can be found in the lumen. They are not absorbed. There is a defect in glucose and galactose transport which was demonstrated by radioautographic labeling of intestinal mucosa incubated with 14C-labeled galactose. The diarrhea responds promptly to replacement of the usual dietary carbohydrates by fructose.

MALADAPTATION SYNDROME

The previously described conditions are all specific inherited enzyme deficiencies, usually with a specific therapy. All are uncommon (with the exception of lactase deficiency). On the other hand, there are many patients with chronic intestinal complaints who have ill-defined dietary intolerances, usually to carbohydrates. In these patients, no specific enzyme defect has as yet been defined, but they often respond to restriction of dietary carbohydrates.

In a series of studies performed over the past decade and reviewed recently (18) Rosensweig and associates demonstrated the adaptive nature of human jejunal glycolytic enzymes as well as disaccharidases to dietary sugars. In general, there is a 100% or more increase in enzyme activities on a high carbohydrate diet as compared to a carbohydrate-free diet. This effect with glycolytic enzymes occurs within 1 day. In addition, they have described a group of patients with chronic gastrointestinal complaints, usually with diarrhea and negative conventional gastrointestinal evaluations, who have a failure of adaptation of the glycolytic enzymes to dietary sugars. Many of these patients are made worse by high carbohydrate diets and are improved by carbohydrate-restricted diets. This condition has been termed an "intestinal maladaptation syndrome." No enzyme deficiency state has been documented. Rather, the authors feel this may represent a failure of the proper regulation of enzyme activity (or metabolism) by normal exogenous factors such as diet. More work is needed to define this condition more exactly.

REFERENCES

1. P. Cuatrecasas, D. H. Lockwood, and J. R. Caldwell, *Lancet,* **1,** 14 (1965).
2. G. T. Keusch, F. J. Troncale, B. Thavaramara, P. Prinyavont, P. R. Anderson, and N. B. Bhamarapiavath, *Am. J. Clin. Nutr.,* **22,** 638 (1969).

96   Carbohydrates

3. T. Gilat, S. Russo, E. Gelman-Malachi, and T. A. M. Aldor, *Gastroenterology,* **62,** 1125 (1972).
4. N. S. Rosensweig, "Intestinal Enzyme Deficiencies and Their Nutritional Implications," *Symposia of the Swedish Nutrition Foundation XI,* 1973, p. 21.
5. K. B. Knudsen, J. D. Welsh, R. S. Kronenberg, et al., *Am. J. Dig. Dis.,* **13,** 593 (1968).
6. N. S. Rosensweig and R. H. Herman, *Am. J. Clin. Nutr.,* **22,** 99 (1969b).
7. M. D. Kogut, G. N. Donnell, and K. N. F. Shaw, *J. Pediat.,* **71,** 75 (1967).
8. N. S. Rosensweig, *Gastroenterology,* **60,** 464 (1971).
9. N. S. Rosensweig and R. H. Herman, *J. Clin. Invest.,* **47,** 2253 (1968).
10. N. S. Rosensweig and R. H. Herman, *Gastroenterology,* **56,** 500 (1969).
11. N. S. Rosensweig and R. H. Herman, *Am. J. Clin. Nutr.,* **23,** 1373 (1970).
12. H. L., Greene, F. B. Stifel, and R. H. Herman, *Biochem. Med.,* **6,** 409 (1972).
13. E. R. Froesch, "Essential Fructosuria and Hereditary Fructose Intolerance," in *The Metabolic Basis of Inherited Disease,* III, McGraw-Hill, N.Y., 1972, p. 141.
14. N. S. Rosensweig, R. H. Herman, F. B. Stifel, and Y. F. Herman, *J. Clin. Invest.,* **48,** 2038 (1969).
15. H. L. Greene, F. B. Stifel, and R. H. Herman, *Clin. Res.,* **20,** 275 (1972) (abstr.).
16. S. Segal, "Disorders of Galactose Metabolism," in *The Metabolic Basis of Inherited Disease,* III, McGraw-Hill, N.Y., 1972, p. 174.
17. G. Meeuwisse, "Enzyme Deficiencies and Their Nutrition Implications," *Symposia of the Swedish Nutrition Foundation XI,* 1973, p. 94.
18. N. S. Rosensweig, *Am. J. Clin. Nutr.,* **28,** 648 (1975).

PART 4

Diabetes

7

The Genetics of
Diabetes Mellitus

JOHN F. NICHOLSON, M.D.

Columbia University, College of Physicians and Surgeons, New York, New York

Although it has been common knowledge for centuries that diabetes tends to occur in families, the application of the principles of Mendelian genetics to diabetes has proved quite difficult.

First of all diabetes mellitus is usually not present at birth. It generally occurs only after the passage of time. For each generation the prevalence of diabetes increases with advancing age. In order to study genetic influence on the development of diabetes mellitus, it was first necessary to deal with the fact that families tend to share not only genes but also environmental events and conditions. Ideal subjects for comparing environmental influences with genetic ones are sets of twins. Identical twins share both genes and environment while nonidentical twins share a common environment but are genetically only siblings. In an early study, White and Pincus found that concordance for diabetes mellitus was much greater in identical twins than in nonidentical twins (Fig. 1) (1). The significance of the association between diabetes and identity of twins is obviously very great, establishing the importance of genetic influence on the development of diabetes mellitus.

In their study, however, White and Pincus did not specify the clinical type of diabetes mellitus. This omission does not invalidate the conclusion that genetic influences are important but does sidestep the second major problem in the genetic analysis of diabetes mellitus.

In general terms there are two clinical forms of diabetes mellitus (Fig. 2). One commonly known as juvenile-onset, or growth-onset, diabetes is characterized by its occurrence in young individuals with normal habitus, by severe hyperglycemia, ketoacidosis, and a requirement for insulin therapy, and by the absence of complications at the onset of the

99

DIABETES MELLITUS IN TWINS

		DIABETES IN BOTH	
		YES	NO
TWINS	YES	16	17
IDENTICAL	NO	2	61

Figure 1. Comparison of identical and nonidentical twins with respect to concordance for diabetes mellitus (1).

disease. The second clinical form, adult-onset, or maturity-onset, diabetes is characterized by its occurrence in older individuals with obese habitus, by less severe hyperglycemia, absence of ketosis, and absence of an insulin requirement, and by the presence of complications at the time of clinical recognition of the disease. These two clinical forms constitute the ends of a spectrum and in the average diabetes clinic, there are substantial numbers of patients who do not fall easily into one category or another. Given this area of uncertainty, genetic analysis must take into account the possibility that diabetes mellitus is not a single disease. To this point, Cammidge, who was both a geneticist and a diabetologist, examined family histories of patients in his clinic and suggested in 1928 and again in 1934 that in some families with the mild form of diabetes mellitus—the adult-onset variety—he could discern patterns of incidence consistent with dominant inheritance, whereas family histories of some patients with juvenile-onset diabetes mellitus suggested recessive inheritance (2,3). Over the next three decades more elaborate studies, some including glucose tolerance tests, were performed without answering conclusively either whether the two clinical forms of diabetes mellitus are identical or whether they are dominant or recessive. Some forty years after Cammidge's work, Tattersall and Fajans performed their very important study on an unusual group of diabetic subjects, those who have in early life a disorder which is clinically mild, maturity-onset diabetes of the young (MODY) (4). In their comparison of families with juvenile-onset diabetes mellitus (JDM) and those with

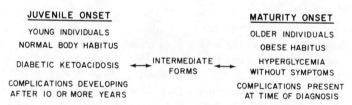

CLINICAL FORMS OF DIABETES MELLITUS

JUVENILE ONSET		MATURITY ONSET
YOUNG INDIVIDUALS		OLDER INDIVIDUALS
NORMAL BODY HABITUS		OBESE HABITUS
DIABETIC KETOACIDOSIS	← INTERMEDIATE → FORMS	HYPERGLYCEMIA WITHOUT SYMPTOMS
COMPLICATIONS DEVELOPING AFTER 10 OR MORE YEARS		COMPLICATIONS PRESENT AT TIME OF DIAGNOSIS

Figure 2. Clinical forms of diabetes mellitus.

MODY they found that 10.8% of the siblings of JDM propositi had diabetes while 44.6% of the siblings of MODY propositi had diabetes. Furthermore, in 85% of the families with MODY a parent had diabetes, and in 44% of these families diabetes was present in three generations. In a number of instances the disease could be shown to be present in four generations (5). Because almost 50% of the siblings of the propositi were found to be diabetic, it is tempting to consider MODY dominantly inherited, but before doing so it is necessary to consider the possibility of recessive inheritance masquerading as dominant inheritance.

In Figure 3, dominance (D) for diabetes is contrasted with the phenomenon of pseudodominance in which a recessive gene for diabetes (d) might appear to be dominant. The cross ND × ND gives rise to offspring 50% of whom are diabetic. If, however, diabetes were inherited as a recessive character and by chance a diabetic subject's mate were a carrier, the resultant cross dd × Nd would give rise to offspring 50% of whom would be diabetic. While pseudodominance can explain the occurrence of a recessive disorder in two generations, this phenomenon is dependent on the accidental mating of a carrier with an affected individual, and is unlikely to explain apparent dominance in three or more generations. It is therefore critical that in 85% of the families studied by Tattersall and Fajans three generations could be shown to be affected and that in some families the disease could be shown to be present in four generations. Furthermore, the disease bred true—the clinical form of diabetes was mild in every generation. Therefore, both the clinical data and the genetic data lead us to accept Tattersall and Fajan's conclusion that maturity-onset diabetes of the young is inherited as an autosomal dominant disorder with virtually complete penetrance.

The next significant advance again concerned diabetes mellitus in the young, but this time the studies involved the severe classic juvenile diabetes mellitus (JDM). A description of these genetic investigations in

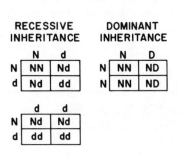

RECESSIVE INHERITANCE

	N	d
N	NN	Nd
d	Nd	dd

	d	d
N	Nd	Nd
d	dd	dd

DOMINANT INHERITANCE

	N	D
N	NN	ND
N	NN	ND

Figure 3. Recessive inheritance (Na × Nd and Nd × dd) and dominant inheritance (ND × NN). D is dominant gene and d is recessive gene for diabetes mellitus.

JDM requires a brief review of the human lymphocyte-associated (HLA) antigen system.

These antigens are genetically determined proteins located on the surfaces of cells, particularly on the surfaces of lymphocytes. Hence the name human lymphocyte-associated antigens. There are four genetic loci for the HLA antigens, HLA-A, HLA-B, HLA-C, and HLA-D. HLA-D is also known as the MLC locus, because it can be detected using the technique of mixed lymphocyte culture. Since the HLA genes are autosomal, each cell has two functioning genes for each of the four loci, and has the capacity to synthesize eight separate antigens. Each HLA locus has many alleles, meaning that an HLA gene can code for any one of many different protein antigens. For comparison's sake, consider the major blood group locus. The gene at this locus can code for any one of the three antigens A, B, and O. Since each cell has two major blood group genes, there are six possible genotypes: AA, AO, AB, BB, BO, and CO. Because of the many different alleles at each HLA locus, and because each cell can synthesize eight separate antigens, the possible HLA genotypes run literally into the tens of thousands and more than 10,000 genotypes have actually been demonstrated. Even though the HLA genes all occur on a relatively small segment of a single chromosome, one would expect to find random combinations of the various alleles. In practice one does not find this. For example, HLA-A1, HLA-B8, and HLA-Dw3 tend to be linked together on the same chromosome more often than one would expect on the basis of random distribution. The same is true for HLA-A2, HLA-B7, and HLA-Dw2. This nonrandomness is called linkage disequilibrium. Since the HLA region has a great deal to do with immune function, and therefore presumably with diseases having to do with immune function, it was reasonable to ask, "Can susceptibilities to certain diseases be treated as genetic functions of the HLA region in linkage disequilibrium with certain specific HLA genes?" In the initial search for this kind of linkage, a spectacular association was discovered between HLA-Bw27 and a disease called ankylosing spondylitis. The overwhelming majority of Caucasians who have ankylosing spondylitis have HLA-Bw27, and the association is so great that the risk of an HLA-Bw27-positive individual's developing the disease is 120 times the risk in the general population (6).

Diabetes mellitus in general showed no specific HLA associations in the early studies, but when the patients were divided into insulin requiring and noninsulin requiring groups, the insulin requiring group showed a rather strong association with HLA-B8, HLA-Bw15, and HLA-Dw3 (7). In studying siblings of juvenile diabetics, Cudworth and

Woodrow noted that when two sibs were both diabetic, they tended to be identical for HLA genes (8).

With this background, Drs. Nicole Suciu-Foca, Pablo Rubinstein, and I embarked on a study of the inheritance of HLA genes in families in which one or more children have juvenile diabetes (9). We required that the propositus, the first child in the family to develop diabetes, need insulin therapy before the age of 10 years, or show evidence of diabetic ketoacidosis, and in any case, be under 16 years of age at the time of diagnosis. We did this to ensure that we would be dealing only with classic juvenile diabetes mellitus and not with some other diabetes syndrome such as MODY. In our study we asked, "What is the relationship of the HLA genes of the siblings of the diabetic propositus to their status with respect to diabetes?" As shown in Figure 3, it is clear that most of the siblings who are diabetic share both HLA-D genes with the propositus. A few do not and in one family the two diabetic siblings do not share any HLA-D genes. Mathematically, however, the evidence is overwhelming that HLA-D identity—that is, sharing both HLA-D genes with the diabetic propositus—defines predisposition for juvenile diabetes mellitus. It is also clear that being identical for HLA-D with a diabetic sibling is not sufficient to make one diabetic (Fig. 3). This observation is not new, since Tattersall and Pyke showed some years ago that only one-half of identical twins of juvenile diabetics develop diabetes (10). Our figures for HLA-D identical siblings of diabetic propositi show that very nearly 50% have diabetes, suggesting that the HLA-D-linked predisposition is sufficient to explain completely the genetic aspect of juvenile diabetes.

The genetic evidence, then, indicates a strong HLA-linked predisposition for juvenile diabetes, which would appear to be necessary, but not sufficient in itself, for the production of the disease.

In genetic terms, juvenile diabetes shows incomplete penetrance in that only a fraction of those carrying the genes for diabetes actually become diabetic. Since identical twins are probably not more likely to share diabetes than are HLA-identical siblings, it is unlikely that genes other than HLA genes precipitate the disease in susceptible individuals. Therefore, juvenile diabetes is actually an acquired disease that is limited to a genetically susceptible population. Several lines of evidence and speculation point to a virus (or viruses) as the actual cause of juvenile diabetes mellitus. For example, juvenile diabetes mellitus tends to occur in outbreaks and shows a seasonal incidence similar to that of viral epidemics (11). Although no specific virus can be pointed to with certainty as the responsible agent, epidemiologic data have incriminated both mumps virus and coxsackie B4 (12,13). Moreover in the few children who have died shortly after the onset of diabetes, inflammatory changes have been shown in the islets of Langerhans that are compatible with an immune response linked to a viral infection (14). Now the HLA region in man is analogous to the H-2 genetic region of the mouse, which is known to be instrumental in determining the mouse's immune response to some viruses. One can therefore speculate that an HLA-linked immune response in man could, for example, be inadequate to prevent viral destruction of the beta cells. On the other hand, an HLA-linked immune response to a viral challenge might itself destroy beta cells by cross reaction. Such cross reactions could in fact be normal transient responses to certain viruses, but abnormally persistent in individuals genetically predisposed to juvenile diabetes. Whatever the ultimate truth, current thought is that juvenile diabetes mellitus is likely to be the result of a viral infection, but that JDM develops only in those individuals who are genetically susceptible through the inheritance of genes which direct the immune response to the causative virus.

The studies discussed so far have dealt with diabetes mellitus in the young. Family studies in the adult population are more difficult to perform, and information concerning genetic influences on the development of diabetes in adults is therefore less well developed. The following can be said. In a study of identical twins, concordance for adult-onset mild diabetes mellitus was found to approach 100% (10). This finding is compatible with the notion that this form of diabetes is entirely determined by inheritance, as is MODY. Insulin-dependent diabetes mellitus with onset in adult life shows associations with specific HLA antigens similar to those seen in JDM (7). In a recent study of retinopathy in adult-onset diabetes Becker found that patients with retinopathy showed no HLA associations, while those without retinopathy showed the HLA associations seen in JDM (15). Since retinopathy is associated with long-standing diabetes, these results suggest that, in the study population, non-HLA-associated diabetes was of long duration, that is, mild, before clinical recognition, whereas HLA-associated adult diabetes was of brief duration before clinical recognition. Taken altogether, current studies suggest that there are at least two forms of diabetes mellitus in the adult population, analogous to the two forms seen in young people. One can add a third diabetic state in both age groups—diabetes associated with obesity that disappears upon weight reduction.

In closing, I would like to refer again to Cammidge's early survey of his patient population (Fig. 4). He discerned dominant and recessive forms of diabetes mellitus, and we can more easily define these forms in the young age groups. The studies of adult subjects are as yet only sug-

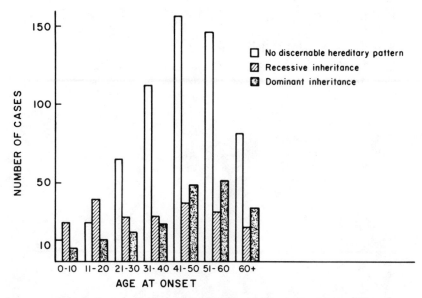

Figure 4.   Genetic anlaysis of 1000 cases of diabetes mellitus (3).

gestive, and now, as then, many patients remain unclassified with respect to the influence of genes on their development of diabetes mellitus. More subdivisions of adult-onset diabetes are entirely possible and in this group, only the outlines of defined genetic influence are as yet visible.

REFERENCES

1.   P. White and G. Pincus, "The etiology and prevention of diabetes, in E. P. Joslin, Ed., *The Treatment of Diabetes Mellitus,* Lea & Febiger, Philadelphia, 1946, p. 57.

2.   P. J. Cammidge, *Brit. Med J.,* **2,** 738 (1928).

3.   P. J. Cammidge, *Lancet,* **1,** 393 (1934).

4.   R. B. Tattersall and S. S. Fajans, *Diabetes,* **24,** 44 (1975).

5.   S. S. Fajans, Personal communication.

6.   A. Svejgaard, P. Platz, L. P. Ryder, L. Staub-Nielsen, and M. Thomsen, *Transplant Rev.,* **22,** 3 (1975).

7.   M. Thomsen, P. Platz, O. O. Andersen, M. Christy, J. Lyngsøe, J. Nerup, K. Rasmussen, L. P. Ryder, L. S. Nielsen, and A. Svejgaard, *Transplant Rev.,* **22,** 125 (1975).

8.   A. E. Cudworth and J. C. Woodrow, *Brit. Med. J.,* **3,** 133 (1975).

9. P. Rubinstein, N. Suciu-Foca, and J. F. Nicholson, *N. Engl. J. Med.*, **297**, 1036 (1977).

10. R. B. Tattersall and D. A. Pyke, *Lancet*, **2**, 1120 (1972).

11. D. R. Gamble and K. W. Taylor, *Brit. Med. J.*, **3**, 631 (1969).

12. D. R. Gamble, M. L. Kinsley, M. G. Fitzgerald, R. Bolton, and K. W. Taylor, *Brit. Med. J.*, **3**, 627 (1969).

13. H. B. Sultz, B. A. Hart, M. Zielezny, and E. R. Schlesinger, *J. Pediat.*, **86**, 654 (1975).

14. W. Gepts, *Diabetes*, **14**, 619 (1965).

15. B. Becker, D. H. Shin, D. Burgess, C. Kilo, and W. V. Miller, *Diabetes*, **26**, 998 (1977).

8

Nutritional Management of
Adult and Juvenile Diabetics

EDWIN L. BIERMAN, M.D.

University of Washington, School of Medicine, Seattle, Washington

We have recently begun to understand the genetic basis for the various, distinct clinical types of diabetes that exist in man. In particular, it is now appreciated that a multiplicity of inherited disorders may be associated with diabetes mellitus. Despite this variation in genetic types, information regarding the best nutritional management of the different forms of clinical diabetes has been available (1) and is adapted to today's knowledge. Dietary approaches, like other forms of therapy, are continually being modified as our understanding increases.

About a decade ago a monumental effort, the UGDP study, explored the question of the effects of treatment of diabetes with oral agents, with regard to morbidity and mortality outcomes. Results of this study have been controversial with regard to the use of oral agents in the management of diabetes. However, one conclusion of that study which did not arouse much controversy was that "diet alone" is the cornerstone of treatment of diabetes in man (2). Therefore, one is entitled to ask the question: what is diet alone?

One can ask the diabetic—the National Health Survey in 1968 did exactly that. Diabetics were surveyed to learn something about their understanding of their own dietary management. One-quarter of the diabetic respondees were never given a diet. Another quarter received the diet but did not follow it. The remaining half followed a diet given to them by their physicians but when questioned further, most failed to understand it.

One is entitled to ask the physician: what is a diabetic diet? About fifty physicians in the Seattle area were surveyed (3), given a hypothetical 19-year-old male who was a diabetic with specific laboratory findings, the classical type of juvenile diabetic discussed in Chapter 7. Fourteen physicians gave him 1 g of protein per kilo of body weight each day, eight others thought 2 g would do, four cut the allowance down to ½ g of protein, and five rather liberal physicians said that protein intake could be unrestricted. For this same patient, five physicians prescribed a total daily calorie allowance of 1000, six others said he could have 1500 calories, nine thought 2000 calories would be just fine, while the remaining five threw caution to the winds and allowed the boy 2500 calories. When it comes to regulating carbohydrate intake for a diabetic, one would expect one's colleagues to be consistent. They were not. Each had only the bare diagnostic facts upon which to base his opinion, but the same facts meant different things to different doctors. Three said our diabetic should have no more than 100 g of carbohydrates a day, seven said 150 g were acceptable, nine pushed the allowance to 200, two specified 225, and one respondant allowed the patient 250 g of carbohydrate each day. There was no correlation between the amount of carbohydrate the boy was allowed and the number of calories permitted. So clearly our understanding of "diet alone" as the cornerstone of management of diabetes leaves much to be desired. Neither the patient nor the physician understands it.

To understand the diabetic diet, an agreement must be reached regarding its goals. The objectives of control of diabetes in general, not just with diet, can be idealized (Table 1). Ideal objectives include prevention of macrovascular disease (i.e., atherosclerotic sequellae, coronary artery disease, and peripheral vascular disease), prevention of microvascular disease, the capillary microangiopathy manifest as eye disease (retinopathy) or kidney disease (nephropathy), and prevention of the nerve deterioration in diabetes (neuropathy).

From a practical point of view, there are objectives of control of blood glucose in diabetes that can actually be achieved by treatment, although

Table 1   Objectives of Control of Blood Glucose: Ideal

1. Prevent macrovascular disease
   Atherosclerotic coronary artery disease
   Peripheral vascular disease

2. Prevent microvascular disease
   Retinopathy
   Nephropathy

3. Prevent neuropathy

Table 2   Objectives of Control of Blood Glucose: Practical

1. Prevent polyuria, vaginitis
2. Prevent hyperosmolar coma
3. Prevent ketoacidosis and coma
4. Reduce hypertriglyceridemia
5. Avoid hypoglycemia

far from the ideal (Table 2). Thus, practically, prevention of the symptoms of uncontrolled diabetes, vaginitis, hyperosmolar coma (a result of severe dehydration and hyperglycemia), ketoacidosis, and coma, can be achieved with insulin treatment. Hypertriglyceridemia also can be reduced. Clearly, the caveat in the regulation of blood glucose by treatment is that hypoglycemia, which can be potentially more harmful than hyperglycemia, must be avoided.

Which of these objectives can be accomplished by diet? Some manifestations of the disorder can be altered by diet (Table 3). These include reversion to normal of plasma glucose levels, urine glucose excretion, plasma lipid (cholesterol and triglyceride) levels, and body weight. The most interesting and probably the most potentially effective dietary maneuver is caloric restriction to effect weight reduction, since with successful caloric restriction all the other abnormalities affected by diet will normalize, that is, elevated plasma glucose levels will be reduced, glycosuria will be eliminated, and plasma cholesterol and triglyceride levels will be lowered. Thus, of these parameters that can actually be changed by diet, weight reduction by diet becomes a most logical goal, particularly since most adult diabetics are obese (4). Also epidemiologic studies (5) show that in many countries the higher the average body weight of the population, the greater the prevalence of diabetes in the country.

Table 3   Manifestations of Diabetes Potentially Influenced by Dietary Management

Hyperglycemia
Glycosuria
Hypercholesterolemia
Hypertriglyceridemia
Obesity

It has long been known that the abnormal glucose tolerance characteristic of obese diabetics can be normalized simply by weight reduction (6). Weight reduction and maintenance of a new lower weight leads to reduction of elevated plasma cholesterol and triglyceride levels (7). Thus, caloric restriction is the underpinning and the primary goal in the management of the adult obese diabetic. Unfortunately, many individuals have equated diabetes with caloric restriction, which has led to growth retardation in many juvenile diabetics who are not given sufficient calories for normal growth and development. This is a particular problem in conjunction with insulin-dependent diabetes, where nutritional deficiencies are more prevalent and it is more difficult to obtain optimum nutritional management.

Therefore, diet therapy in diabetes mellitus is concerned primarily with total calories—calorie restriction in the adult diabetic and the provision of adequate calories to maintain normal growth and development in the insulin-dependent juvenile diabetic. The MODY group (maturity-onset diabetes in the young) described in Chapter 7 should be treated like adult diabetics except that, since the disorder occurs before the age of 30, sufficient calories should be given for normal growth and development, and special attention should be paid to the prevention of overweight.

The timing of meals is particularly important to the juvenile-onset insulin-dependent diabetic receiving long-acting insulin as subcutaneous injections one or more times during the day. Clearly, without a normally functioning endocrine pancreas, the minute-to-minute regulation of blood glucose by pancreatic hormones needed to modulate periods of feeding and fasting is absent. Ingestion of meals to match the injections of insulin is appropriate, and thus a diabetic must partake of at least 5 feedings a day, if not more. No period of more than 3 to 4 hours without food during the waking day is a very important pattern of dietary intake for the prevention of hypoglycemia, which when frequent and severe can lead to more devastating complications than hyperglycemia, particularly in terms of nervous system and brain function.

The composition of the diabetic diet is potentially the most controversial area of concern. Should the proportion of fat and carbohydrate in the diabetic diet be altered with regard to effects on glucose homeostasis and long-term vascular complications? The history of the composition of the diabetic diet is somewhat checkered (Table 4) (8). Before the insulin era, diet therapy uniformly consisted of low calories, for example, the "fast days" of Allen, but the carbohydrate content recommended was either high or low in proportion to the rest of the

Table 4   History of Dietary Composition (Relative Proportion of Carbohydrate and Fat Calories) Used in Management of Diabetes Mellitus

Date	Source	Carbohydrate	Fat
1550 B.C. (approx.)	Ebers papyrus (Egypt)	High	
0001	Aretaeus (Asia Minor)	High	
1675	Willis	High	
1797	Rollo	Very low	High
1860–80	Bouchardat	Low	High
1900–1920	Naunyn; Allen	Low (+ fasting)	Low
1900–1920	von Noorden	High	
1923	Geyelin	High	
1929	Sansum	Normal	Normal
1931	Rabinowitch	Moderate	Low
1935	Himsworth	High	
1940–60	Kempner; Ernest	High	Low
1940–70	A.D.A. (U.S.)	Limited	Moderate
1971 to date	A.D.A. (U.S.)	Increased	Reduced

calories. As a rule, the cause of death was ketoacidosis when patients became deficient in insulin. But there were physicians, like Rollo and Bouchardat, who claimed that restricting carbohydrate drastically helped during the time before patients became overtly insulin deficient. And there were others who referred to "high carbohydrate cures," for example, the "oatmeal diet" of von Noorden. This controversy should have been laid to rest in 1921 after the discovery of insulin, when it was possible to give a normal diet as long as sufficient insulin was given to help metabolize dietary macronutrients. The object of diet therapy, after insulin was discovered, was to maintain an ideal body weight by giving insulin and modulating calories. But again there was controversy as to whether carbohydrate content should be relatively high or low. The major cause of death now in the "insulin era" is not ketoacidosis, but atherosclerosis. More than two-thirds of diabetics today die of one or more complications of atherosclerosis, most often coronary artery disease (9). In terms of the ultimate goal of diet therapy this fact should certainly be kept in mind. Many physicians in the 1920s and even in the early 1930s reported on the use of normal or even high carbohydrate diets, giving sufficient insulin simultaneously. However, alternative views promoting carbohydrate-restricted diets seemed to hold sway. As Glick wrote in the *New England Journal of Medicine* in 1971 in a letter to the editor (10), referring to the amount of space devoted to the "high carbohydrate theory" in different editions of Joslin's textbook *Diabetes,*

"The number of pages assigned to this theory rose to a maximum of 6 ½ in the fifth (1935), and sixth (1937) editions, fell to three pages in the seventh (1940), was demoted to an italicized section in the eighth edition (1946), and disappeared completely in the ninth edition (1952), and thereafter." Glick likens the disappearance of the high carbohydrate diet without a trace to the fate that befell theories at variance with the party line in successive editions of the Russian encyclopedia.

Where does this leave us in terms of the evidence upon which to base a conclusion about the best way to approach the macronutrient composition of the optimal diabetic diet? If we examine the problem of the risk for atherosclerosis in the diabetic, it is clear that the diabetic suffers from the same risk factors prevalent in the general population, except that most are magnified (Table 5) (11). Hyperglycemia is more prevalent in the diabetic by definition. At least one-third of treated diabetic populations have one or more forms of hyperlipidemia. There appears to be more hypertension in the diabetic, perhaps because there is more obesity, but possibly because of other factors as well. Obesity is far more prevalent in the diabetic. The question of the role of dietary fat versus carbohydrate is of interest. Traditionally, in the last 30 years (Table 4) the diabetic diet given in many instances was a high fat, high cholesterol diet, and this type of diet has been thought by some to be a risk factor for atherogenesis. Diabetics tend to have high circulating insulin levels, whether in the obese adult diabetic who has hyperinsulinism as a result of obesity, or in the insulin-treated young diabetic because of the inability to regulate precisely the amount of insulin needed in the blood at a particular time. During the 24-hour period, the insulin-treated diabetic may often have high insulin levels. Thus the arterial wall may be

Table 5   Risk Factors for Atherosclerosis in Diabetes

Risk Factor	General Population	Diabetics
Hyperglycemia	+	+++
Hypertriglyceridemia	++	+++
Hypercholesterolemia	++	+++
Hypertension	++	+++
Hyperinsulinemia	+	++
Obesity	+	+++
Dietary fat and cholesterol	+	++
Cigarette smoking	+++	+++
Genetic factors	?	?

bathed at times with high insulin levels in all forms of diabetes. This might contribute to altered metabolism of the arterial wall as well as to higher lipoprotein levels in the circulation. Finally, there are genetic factors that are not yet understood, particularly since we are only now beginning to understand the genetic basis of diabetes. Perhaps one of the genetic manifestations of the disorder might be a cellular defect affecting the arterial wall and predisposing to atherosclerosis.

Early evidence relating to the effect of dietary carbohydrate on glucose metabolism was provided in 1935 by Himsworth (12). This information is still valid and in fact has been periodically rediscovered. Young healthy volunteers were placed on a series of diets, varied only in the amount of carbohydrate, which was substituted for fats isocalorically. The diets contained from 50 g to 500 g of carbohydrate; glucose tolerance tests were performed on each diet. The higher the amount of carbohydrate in the diet the better the glucose tolerance, almost as a continuous function. This information has been used repeatedly by physicians who do glucose tolerance testing and give a minimum of 300 g of carbohydrate in the diet to ensure that "starvation diabetes" as a result of carbohydrate restriction is avoided. In other words, with severe carbohydrate restriction, abnormal glucose tolerance results. However, 300 g of carbohydrate is an arbitrary figure. The higher the carbohydrate intake, the better the glucose tolerance.

In the 1970s this "Himsworth phenomenon" was rediscovered by Anderson (13), who did similar experiments, albeit somewhat more precisely as can be done today in a metabolic ward using liquid formula diets of constant composition. In his studies, glucose or sucrose was the only source of carbohydrate in formulas ranging from 20% carbohydrate to 80% carbohydrate as isocaloric substitutions for fat. Again there was a continuous improvement in glucose tolerance in normal volunteer subjects as the proportion of carbohydrate in the diet was increased. A possible mechanism that still holds today was suggested by Himsworth using intravenous insulin injections and following how rapidly and how much the blood glucose declines. On the different diets of varying carbohydrate composition, the higher the carbohydrate, the more glucose disappears from the blood stream. It has been noted elsewhere in this volume that, at least in the intestinal wall, higher carbohydrate diets lead to enzyme adaptation for better metabolism of glucose. This is true not only in the intestinal wall, but also in muscle tissue, in adipose tissue, and apparently in all tissues involved in glucose utilization and metabolism. This is an adaptive response to higher carbohydrate diets such that glucose is used more efficiently. In our laboratory, Brunzell (14) studied mild adult-onset obese diabetics on a metabolic ward. Compared with a basal 45% carbohydrate diet, on an 85% dextrose diet glucose tolerance improved even in mild diabetics. Most of this improvement appeared to be in the fasting glucose level. The rapidity of glucose disappearance from the blood in response to intravenous insulin was also measured. In most of the subjects on the higher carbohydrate diet, even in mild diabetics, glucose disappearance was accelerated, confirming Himsworth's earlier results.

The source of dietary carbohydrate or type of sugar does not seem to influence results. Dunnigan showed that fasting blood glucose levels were similar whether on a sucrose-free diet or a diet containing sucrose as the source of carbohydrate (15). Anderson documented improved glucose tolerance in normal subjects on 80% sucrose diets (13).

Brunzell extended these studies from mild diabetics to treated diabetics who were maintained on insulin or oral antidiabetic therapy (16). With the same dietary protocol, when basal (40%) carbohydrate was compared to high (85%) carbohydrate (as dextrose), treated diabetics, whether on insulin or on oral agents, all lowered their fasting plasma glucose levels on the high carbohydrate diet. Even on extremes of 85% carbohydrate in the diet, as long as these diabetics remained treated there was no increase in 24-hour urinary glucose. However, when the untreated, decompensated diabetic is examined, an inability to handle the extra dietary carbohydrate becomes apparent. On an 85% carbohydrate diet, urinary glucose increased in a group of untreated diabetics. Therefore, high carbohydrate diets can be handled effectively by diabetics as long as there is insulin available, whether given by injection or whether endogenously secreted, such as in the adult obese diabetic. Only when there is no insulin available and the patient is untreated is the diabetic unable to handle dietary carbohydrate.

These data were obtained from metabolic studies, in which extreme dietary perturbations were made to study alterations in metabolism and to better understand the handling of macronutrients. What about practical diets that can be given to diabetics? There are relatively few long-term diet studies that apply to the diabetic. Diabetics usually have been excluded from most diet studies, particularly in relation to atherosclerosis, because they would complicate study design and interpretation. Furthermore, there have been very few studies in which various diets have been tested prospectively, on an outpatient basis, in the management of diabetes. An exception is the 2-year study of Stone and Connor (17) published 15 years ago. They tested the effect of long-term high carbohydrate, low fat diets in diabetics, using more than fifty insulin-requiring young diabetics and two study diets. The control diet was the ADA diet then in use, which contained about 17% of calories as protein, 41% as carbohydrate, and 42% as fat, and contained 900 mg of cholesterol per day. The experimental diet contained the same amount of protein, 64% carbohydrate, and 20% fat, with cholesterol content very restricted to 100 mg. The object of the study was to test whether this diet, which would be very prudent for the prevention of atherosclerosis in diabetics, would be of practical use in the management of young insulin-treated diabetics. On the experimental diet there was no change in weight and no increase in insulin dosage requirement. In fact, in some patients there was a decreased insulin requirement. Some subjects had more hypoglycemic reactions and required a reduction in their insulin doses. We have observed comparable results (unpublished) under similar circumstances. Of note, there was a dramatic decrease in cholesterol levels and a decrease in fasting triglyceride levels on the high carbohydrate, low fat diet. The conclusion of Stone and Connor's study was that there was no obvious deleterious effect of such a diet, during the short term of 2 years, and perhaps a beneficial effect with regard to hyperlipidemia and the prevention of the premature and severe atherosclerosis to which diabetics are so prone. These conclusions were largely confirmed by Weinsier et al. (18) in a study of 18 diabetics not requiring insulin comparing 40% and 55% carbohydrate isocaloric diets. In contrast to these studies, there have been no comparable controlled studies of a low carbohydrate diet in diabetes. In every study which reportedly tested a low carbohydrate diet, the diet was also a low calorie diet because carbohydrate and calories were restricted simultaneously. Since calorie restriction is so potent in reversing all of the metabolic abnormalities of the adult obese diabetic, the answer to the question about the efficacy of a disproportionately low carbohydrate isocaloric diet remains unknown.

There is a high prevalence of elevated plasma lipid levels in garden variety treated diabetics, studied in clinic populations. In one such study (19) triglyceride levels were elevated in adult diabetics but not in juvenile diabetics; cholesterol levels were elevated in adult diabetics but *also* in juvenile diabetics. This trend to hypercholesterolemia in young diabetics appeared very puzzling until a study by Kaufman (20) helped to clarify the problem. Diabetic children in a summer camp were studied, with a focus on the question of whether hypercholesterolemia in the young diabetic results from the diets commonly prescribed. The usual diabetic diet contained 700 to 1500 mg a day of cholesterol with a polyunsaturated:saturated fat ratio of 0.1; the study diet was modified in such a way as to reduce its cholesterol content to the moderate 300 mg a day, with a P:S ratio of 1.0, which is the current American Heart Association dietary recommendation. These children were fed the diets controlled from the camp kitchen in random order. On both diets triglyceride levels, which were slightly elevated, fell. Since triglyceride levels are responsive to changes in insulin management, it was clear that these diabetic children were managed more closely while they were in camp; hence the reduction in triglyceride levels. However, on the usual diet, cholesterol levels were elevated for children of this age and they remained elevated throughout maintenance on their usual diet. However, when fed the low cholesterol, low saturated fat diet, their cholesterol levels were lowered to the normal range seen in nondiabetic children. The strong suggestion from the results of this study is that the hypercholesterolemia that has been observed in young diabetics may have been the result of inappropriate diabetic dietary management, that is, carbohydrate restriction resulting in high fat and high cholesterol diets.

Some adult diabetic patients also have one of the familial forms of hypertriglyceridemia, which can be a risk factor associated with atherosclerosis. In such individuals, basal triglyceride levels may rise in response to increases in dietary carbohydrate. However, since most diabetics are obese, hypertriglyceridemia, when present, responds to caloric restriction as in nondiabetic patients. Recent attention to plasma levels of glucose and triglyceride throughout the 24-hour period indicates that triglyceride levels may actually decrease during the day on higher carbohydrate diets while postprandial glucose levels are increased (21).

Current understanding thus leads to a basic dietary approach for the diabetic (Table 6). This is fundamentally a low calorie diet, which applies mainly to the adult diabetic who is usually obese. This approach is not appropriate for the young diabetic who needs adequate calories. For both types of diabetes, a low saturated fat, low cholesterol diet is recommended, which translates into substitution of carbohydrate for fat. The role of fiber and various natural sugars in the nutritional management of diabetes is currently under investigation.

This diet is a reasonable one not only for the diabetic; it is also a conceptually practical unified single diet approach for the treatment of the individual with hyperlipidemia. In fact, it is a prudent dietary approach for the general population as a whole. This diet is nontoxic, since noth-

Table 6   The Basic Diet

Low calorie
Low saturated fat
Low cholesterol

ing is added, and it has the advantage of reversing obesity, hypercholesterolemia, hypertriglyceridemia, and hyperglycemia, all potentially harmful consequences of the diabetic state.

REFERENCES

1. E. L. Bierman, et al., *Diabetes,* **20,** 633, (1971).
2. University Group Diabetes Program, *Diabetes,* **19,** (suppl 2) (1970).
3. R. H. Barnes, *Nutr. Today,* September 1968, pp 21–25.
4. *Joslin's Diabetes Mellitus,* A. Marble, Ed., 11th ed., Lea & Febiger, Philadelphia, 1971.
5. K. M. West and J. M. Kalbfliesch, *Diabetes,* **20,** 99 (1971).
6. L. H. Newburgh and J. W. Conn, *J.A.M.A.,* **112,** 7 (1939).
7. J. Olefsky, G. M. Reaven, and J. W. Farquhar, *J. Clin. Invest.,* **53,** 64 (1974).
8. F. C. Wood, Jr., and E. L. Bierman, *Nutr. Today,* May/June, 1972, pp. 4–12.
9. H. H. Marks and L. F. Krall, In: *Joslin's Diabetes Mellitus,* A. Marble, Ed., Lea & Febiger, Philadelphia, 1971, pp. 209–54.
10. S. Glick, *New Engl. J. Med.,* **285,** 58 (1971).
11. E. L. Bierman and J. D. Brunzell, In *Advances in Modern Nutrition,* Vol. 2., H. M. Katzen and R. J. Mahler, Eds., Wiley, New York, 1978.
12. H. P. Himsworth, *Clin. Sci.,* **2,** 67 (1935).
13. J. A. Anderson, R. H. Herman, and D. Zakim, *Am. J. Clin. Nutr.,* **26,** 600 (1973).
14. J. D. Brunzell, R. L. Lerner, W. R. Hazzard, D. Porte, Jr., and E. L. Bierman, *New Engl. J. Med.,* **284,** 521 (1971).
15. M. G. Dunningan, T. Fyfe, M. T. McKiddie, and S. M. Crosbie, *Clin. Sci.,* **38,** 1 (1970).
16. J. D. Brunzell, R. L. Lerner, D. Porte, Jr., and E. L. Bierman, *Diabetes,* **23,** 138 (1974).
17. D. B. Stone and W. E. Connor, *Diabetes,* **12,** 127 (1963).
18. R. L. Weinsier, A. Seeman, M. G. Herrera, J. P. Assal, J. S. Soeldner, and R. E. Gleason, *Ann. Int. Med.,* **80,** 332 (1974).
19. M. I. New, T. N. Roberts, E. L. Bierman, and G. G. Reader, *Diabetes,* **12,** 208 (1963).
20. R. L. Kaufman, J. P. Assal, J. S. Soeldner, E. G. Wilmhurst, J. R. Lemaire, R. E. Gleason, and P. White, *Diabetes,* **24,** 672 (1975).
21. G. Schlierf, W. Reinheimer, and V. Stossberg, *Nutr. Metab.,* **13,** 80 (1971).

9

Dietary Management of the Pregnant Diabetic

ROBERT H. KNOPP, M.D., MARIAN T. CHILDS,
PH.D., and MARIA R. WARTH, M.D.

The Northwest Lipid Research Clinic, Harborview Medical Center, and the
Department of Medicine, University of Washington Medical School, Seattle,
Washington

The diet of the pregnant diabetic must serve two needs, the glycemic control of the mother and the nutritional needs of the fetus. In the attempt to achieve glycemic control, diabetic diets differ, depending on the kind of diabetes a person has (1,2). Distribution of dietary carbohydrate throughout the day to complement the effect of insulin and to minimize hyperglycemic and hypoglycemic swings is the primary objective in the normal weight, insulin requiring, ketosis prone, unstable diabetic. Caloric restriction and enhancement of the effectiveness of the available endogenous insulin are the prime objectives in the treatment of the usually obese, noninsulin requiring, ketosis-resistant, stable diabetic.

To meet the nutritional needs of the fetus, there must be sufficient increments in all nutrients. There is general agreement on the additional amounts of protein, vitamins, and minerals that should be allowed in the pregnancy diet (3). However, there has been debate on the question of maternal calorie intake and the restriction of dietary carbohydrate and fat. The National Academy of Sciences Food and Nutrition Board (4) and others (3,5) have recommended an ample maternal calorie intake and weight gain in normal pregnancy.

The need for optimal nutrient supply to the fetus comes into direct conflict with the need for glycemic control in the mother when caloric restriction is seen as the prime treatment mode in the pregnant diabetic. Opinions of various authorities on caloric restriction as an objective in treating the pregnant diabetic vary widely from categorical limitation in

119

weight gain (6), to caloric restriction only in the obese pregnant diabetic (7), or no comment at all on the question (8,9), to a reasonable awareness of the problem (10,11).

The precise way in which ample food intake and consequent maternal weight gain minimize fetal mortality and morbidity is not known. The objectives of this chapter are to examine the available data on caloric requirement and regulation of maternal weight gain in normal and diabetic pregnancy, to assess effects of altered diet composition in pregnancy, and to formulate guidelines for diet therapy in the diabetic pregnancy.

CONTROL OF MATERNAL VERSUS FETAL WEIGHT GAIN

In the normal pregnancy, it is estimated that about 200 extra kcal daily are required (3). The extra energy may be derived from increased food intake or decreased activity or both, with a net accumulation of approximately 25 lb during the course of gestation (4). The result is a steady weight gain of about 1 lb/week in the last two trimesters, which serves as a continuous record of successful progress in the gestation, and a final average weight gain of about 25 lb.

The approximately linear rate of weight gain in pregnancy has two principal components with different dimensions in time (5). About one-fourth of the weight gain is maternal fat, which accumulates primarily in the first half of gestation. The remaining maternal weight gain is increased plasma volume and the conceptus (fetus, uterus, and attendant fluids and membranes), which accumulate primarily in the second half of gestation.

The determination that the pregnant human gains adipose tissue fat in early gestation is based on the elegant studies of Hytten and co-workers (12). They used deuterium or heavy water as a marker for total body water to calculate the component of maternal weight gain which is largely water free, that is, the adipose tissue fat (12). The pattern of maternal fat gain is illustrated in Figure 1, upper panel. A strikingly similar pattern of adipose tissue fat accumulation is seen in the laboratory rat as seen from total body fatty acid measurements obtained serially throughout gestation by Beaton, Beare, Ryu, and McHenry (13) (Fig. 2, upper panel) and ourselves in serial measurements of lumbar fat pads in the middle and late gestation pregnant rat (Fig. 2, lower panel).

It may be questioned why Seitchik (14) and Emerson and colleagues (15) did not find any evidence for maternal fat accumulation using

METABOLIC CHANGES IN HUMAN PREGNANCY

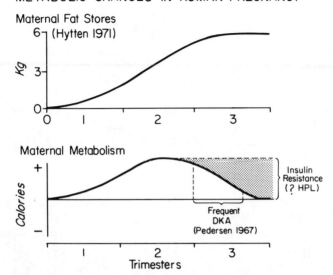

Figure 1. Changes in maternal fat storage. Upper panel shows that maternal fat storage is nearly complete by the end of the second trimester. Lower panel depicts the rate of weight gain which is maximal in midgestation. The decline in the rate of fat storage is associated with the onset of maternal insulin resistance and the time of most frequent occurrence of diabetic ketoacidosis. Curves are based on the data of Hytten and co-workers (5).

methods similar to those of Hytten et al. (12). The results from the three studies are summarized in Table 1. It appears that Hytten's results may be related to the greater weight gain of his women (12) compared to those studied by Emerson (15). Certain biases in Seitchik's method tend to underestimate total body fat; furthermore, different subjects were studied at different time points, making difficult any estimation of serial change in body weight or fluid in pregnancy (14). A reasonable conclusion from these studies is that the amount of fat that a mother gains in pregnancy is a function of her calorie intake.

To test the idea that maternal food intake is an important determinant of the weight gained in early gestation (when conceptus growth is minimal), pregnant rats were fed an amount of food equal to the intake of nonpregnant age matched controls from days 3 to 12 of gestation (Fig. 3). In the pair-fed group there was no augmentation in food intake and no increase in weight gain over the first 12 days of gestation. Weight gain was in fact less than for another serially studied group of rats allowed ad lib access to food (Fig. 3), and at day 12 of

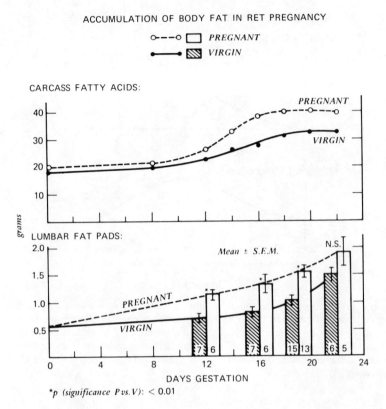

ACCUMULATION OF BODY FAT IN RET PREGNANCY

o---o ☐ *PREGNANT*
●——● ▨ *VIRGIN*

Figure 2.   Changes in maternal fat storage in rat pregnancy. Upper figure shows the accumulation of total body fatty acids according to Beaton et al. (13). Lower figure shows the increase in mass of lumbar fat pads of pregnant and age matched control rats. As rats tend to gain weight with age, the important point is to compare the difference between pregnant and nonpregnant. In both experiments, the increment in fat storage associated with pregnancy is complete by the end of the second gestational week.

gestation was below the 2 SD lower limit for weight gain for six groups of age matched pregnant virgin rat pairs. After day 12, when pair feeding was discontinued, food intake and maternal weight gain increased in the pregnancy group, approaching but never reaching the level of weight gained by the nonpaired pregnant rats (Fig. 3).

The net accumulation of maternal stores may be estimated in pregnant rats of the pair-fed and nonpair-fed experiments by subtracting the average weight of the conceptus (direct weighings obtained from previous observations of ad lib fed rats) and the nonpregnant control rats (Table 2). The results confirm a lesser accumulation of maternal

Table 1   Estimates of Body Fat Gain in Pregnancy[a]

Author	Diet	Weight Gain	Fat Gain
Hytten et al. (75)	To appetite	27.5	7.7
Seitchik (11–40)[b]	Not stated	—[b]	1.1
Emerson et al.			
Normal (5)	Restricted	20.2	↓ in 4, ↑ in 1
Diabetic (2)	Restricted	15.0	↓ in 1, ↑ in 1

[a] Parentheses denote number of subjects studied. Deuterium is administered to determine total body water by the dilution method, allowing nonhydrated body mass (fat) to be calculated. Original references are Hytten et al. (12), Seitchik (14), and Emerson et al. (15).

[b] Based on comparisons of different women at different times in gestation; therefore, weight gain cannot be estimated. The determination of dilution from urinary deuterium underestimates body fat (14) and is probably less accurate than the plasma dilution method used in the other two studies (12,15).

"stores" in the rats pair-fed from days 3 to 12 of gestation. While the nature of the maternal "stores" is not established in these experiments, extracellular fluid volume, fat, and protein all contribute (16). Particularly noteworthy is the decline in these "stores" in late gestation in the nonpair-fed rats which accompanies a pair-fed reduction in food intake in late gestation relative to the pair-fed rats (Table 2, Fig. 3). In the pair-fed rats, a greater food intake in late gestation is apparently sufficient to avoid any net loss of "stores" (Table 2, Fig. 3). These results add further support to the view that maternal fuel storage is closely linked to the level of food intake. The results also suggest that the maternal "stores" may normally be utilized in late gestation. Whether the stores utilized are protein, fat, or both in the rat is not known.

A slight loss in fat stores occurs in the human pregnancy as well between 30 and 38 weeks gestation (data of Hytten et al. (12)). Fat utilization is greatest in the mothers with the greatest degree of overweight prior to pregnancy and the least amount of subsequent fat storage (Table 3) (12). In addition, indirect calorimetry measurements performed by Emerson et al. in human pregnancy support the idea that fat predominates over glucose as a fuel in late gestation (17). These observations justify the conclusion that fat storage in pregnancy serves a nutritional need in late gestation in normal pregnancy as well as in pregnancy where food intake is by chance reduced.

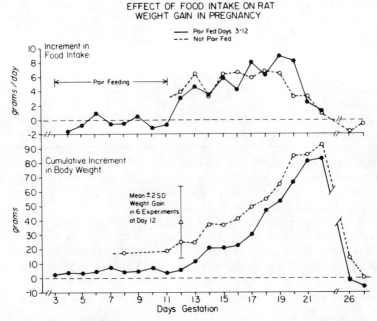

Figure 3. Food restriction and weight gain in rat pregnancy. Rats were fed chow diets and net food intake was measured daily as shown. The pair-fed pregnant rats between gestational days 3 and 12 were fed a diet equal to the amount eaten by age matched nonpregnant rats. The vertical bar denotes the mean ± 2 SD weight increment in six groups of pregnant rats compared to six age matched groups of nonpregnant controls.

Shifts in maternal fuel metabolism accompany the increases in adipose tissue fat accumulation. Figure 4 illustrates the metabolic fate of radio-labeled glucose as a precursor of adipose tissue fat in the pregnant rat model in middle and late gestation (18). It can be seen that de novo glucose conversion into adipose tissue fatty acids in vitro is increased twofold above control in midgestation and reduced to one-third of control in late gestation (Fig. 2, upper panel).

These experiments point to a special adaptation in pregnancy, whereby an energy fuel such as glucose is stored as triglyceride in increased amounts in midgestation and diminished amounts in late gestation. The augmentation of fat stores in midgestation is associated with increased secretion of insulin (18,19), which may reflect increased food intake as well as certain effects of pregnancy hormones.

The diminished utilization of glucose in late gestation may be attributed to an acquired insulin resistance, which has been documented in both late human (19) and late rat pregnancy (20). The insulin resistance is attributed to chorionic somatomammotropin (HCS or placental lactogen), a contrainsulin, lipolytic, polypeptide hormone related to growth hormone but secreted by the placenta in proportion to the rate of growth of the fetal-placental unit (21). Synergism with other pregnancy hormones may also exist (22,23). The temporal relationship between the increasing insulin resistance of late gestation and a declining rate of fat storage is illustrated in Figure 1, lower panel.

Contemporaneous with the increasing insulin antagonism of late gestation are the rising levels of circulating lipid fuels in the form of free fatty acids (see (18) and (19) for review) and triglyceride fatty acids which can serve the energy requirements of maternal tissues such as muscle and uterus. An example of the increase in lipoprotein triglyceride and cholesterol in pregnancy is presented in Table 4. Increased maternal fat oxidation in late gestation was recognized almost 15 years ago by Freinkel as a likely mechanism for sparing maternal glucose for fetal utilization (24), and it is in this sense that Grumbach speaks of HCS as a fetal growth hormone (21).

Table 2   Calculated Composition of Maternal Weight Gain in Pair-Fed and Nonpair-Fed Rats[a]

	Grams			
Gestational Day	12	16	19	21
Pair-fed rats				
Body weight				
Pregnant (7)	233 ± 6[b]	264 ± 7	302 ± 8	331 ± 9
Virgin (7)	227 ± 3	241 ± 3	248 ± 4	249 ± 4
Conceptus weights	3 ± 1[c]	11 ± 2	38 ± 1	66 ± 2
Net maternal gain	3	12	16	16
Nonpair-fed rats				
Body weight				
Pregnant (14)	253 ± 6	272 ± 6	309 ± 7	337 ± 8
Virgin (8)	227 ± 1	230 ± 5	244 ± 9	251 ± 6
Conceptus weights	3 ± 1	11 ± 2	38 ± 1	66 ± 2
Net maternal gain	23	31	27	20

[a] In the pair-fed experiment, the food intake of the pregnant rats was limited to the intake of the nonpregnant animals between days 3 and 12 of gestation.
[b] Mean ± SEM.
[c] Represents 20 to 85 animals at each time in gestation.

Table 3   Body Fat Storage According to
Prior Degree of Obesity in Pregnancy
(12)

| | 10–38 Week Gain (lb) | |
	Total Body Weight	Fat
Light	27.2	6.2
Median	25.3	4.8
Heavy	20.9	1.4

Figure 5 illustrates the shifts in pregnancy fuel metabolism (19b). Early gestation is seen as an anabolic period for both mother and fetus, with relatively slow fetal growth making minimal demands on the mother (Fig. 5-I). In this period, incoming glucose is assimilated in muscle for energy or stored in adipose tissue after being converted to fat. Similarly, circulating triglycerides are stored in increased amounts in adipose tissue. Fat mobilization is limited as glucose adequately meets maternal energy needs and fetal competition for glucose is small. As a result, the maternal adipose tissue store grows (see (19b) for review).

Late gestation is seen as a relatively catabolic period with respect to the mother and a period of increasing anabolism for the rapidly growing fetus (Fig. 5-II). The demand of the fetus for glucose is now much greater. The mother meets this need by appropriately diverting glucose away from her own tissues by the mechanism of insulin resistance, providing alternative substrates for her own tissues in the form of free fatty acids (FFA) or triglycerides. While plasma ketones are usually not increased after an overnight fast (19,25), the pregnant mother is poised to develop ketosis rapidly as a result of the catabolic shift of late gestation should starvation ensue (26,27).

MATERNAL WEIGHT GAIN AND FUEL METABOLISM IN THE DIABETIC PREGNANCY

The changes in the normal pregnant mother may be contrasted with changes that could result from a deficiency of insulin supply from the pancreas or a lack of insulin effectiveness in target tissues. In early gestation, deficient insulin effect would tend to minimize the accumulation of maternal fat, a process known to require insulin. In late gestation, evolving insulin resistance tends to enhance fat mobilization and to prompt ketoacidosis (Fig. 1, lower panel) (28).

Fat metabolism in the insulin treated pregnant diabetic has not been extensively studied. Emerson's studies of six pregnant diabetics by the method of indirect calorimetry (17) suggest that fat is a predominant fuel in late gestation in the diabetic mothers with infants of normal body weight and carbohydrate is the predominant fuel in mothers with large babies and presumably poorer diabetic control. Body fat stores in two pregnant diabetics (deuterium method) (5) accumulated initially, but

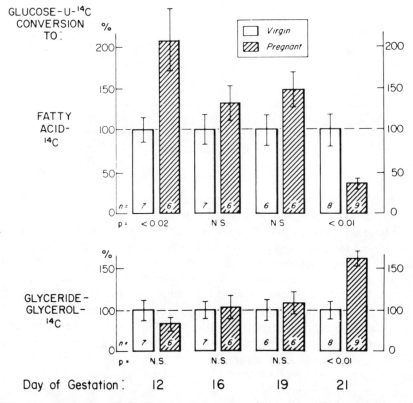

Figure 4. Conversion of glucose into adipose tissue fatty acids and glyceride glycerol in vitro. Compared to control, the peak increase in pregnancy is seen in midgestation (day 12). Lipogenesis then declines to subnormal levels at term. Glucose conversion to glyceride glycerol represents the glucose metabolized to glycerol that is used in re-esterifying fatty acids into their triglyceride storage form. The rate of this process increases as gestation proceeds, corresponding to increased fatty acid mobilization. See (18) for details. Reprinted by permission of the publishers.

Table 4   Serial Blood Lipid Measurements in Subject E. H. in Pregnancy after Overnight Fast

Week[a]	mg/dl					
	5	10	20	29	33	36
Total:						
TG	59	83	147	256	295	276
Chol	154	161	199	217	224	229
VLDL:						
TG	27	40	81	145	200	154
Chol	6	9	15	30	39	38
LDL:						
TG	25	16	39	62	66	84
Chol	92	87	120	132	139	143
HDL:						
TG	9	17	27	34	34	34
Chol	57	59	58	49	46	48
Body weight (kg)	71.8	—	81.0	85.2	86.5	87.5

[a] TG = triglyceride; Chol = cholesterol.

decreased in late gestation, particularly in one subject whose course was complicated by infection, fever, and ketoacidosis.

These data are sufficient to show that an insulin treated diabetic can add to her fat stores during gestation. The greater problem is in the loss of fuel homeostasis per se, that is, exaggerated swings in glucose and lipid fuels, with caloric losses in the form of glycosuria as well as excess caloric deposition in the fetus. As a result, according to Emerson, the diabetic mother's caloric requirement for the whole course of pregnancy is about 5000 kcal higher than it is for the nondiabetic pregnancy (29).

A major unanswered question of diabetic pregnancy is whether weight gain should be encouraged to the same level as in nondiabetic pregnancy, in view of the fact that maternal nutrient supplies to the fetus are already excessive. A major concern related to this question is the development of ketonuria, which is associated with impaired intellectual performance in children of nondiabetic (30,31) as well as diabetic pregnancy (32,33). It is known that limitation of maternal weight gain, whether diabetic or nondiabetic, has the consequence of increasing maternal fatty acid mobilization and ketone body synthesis. There is little evidence that ketonemia or ketonuria is a normal feature of overnight fasting in the adequately fed pregnant mother (19,25), despite the well-documented effect of ketosis on prolonged fasting (26,27). In other words, ketonuria in pregnancy should be regarded as an abnormal phenomenon.

Experience with one pregnant, obese, adult-onset, insulin requiring diabetic is illustrated in Table 5. The patient was given a 1200 kcal ADA diet on an obstetrical ward where her a.m. urines were glucose and ketone free. On transfer to a metabolic ward, the 1200 kcal dietary prescription was continued but was weighed out in a metabolic kitchen. The result was a copious amount of ketonuria (Table 5) despite good control of the diabetes with 50 units of NPH insulin daily. With an increase in her weighed diet to 2000 kcal/day the ketonuria cleared with no deterioration in control of the circulating fuels. The lesson from this case is that prevention of ketonuria in the pregnant diabetic requires an adequate dietary intake to at least maintain calorie balance, just as in the nonpregnant diabetic.

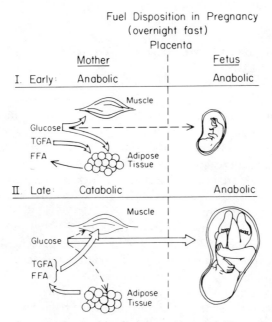

Figure 5. Fuel disposition in pregnancy. The upper panel (I) represents early gestation; the lower panel (II), late gestation. In early gestation, glucose is visualized as the primary maternal metabolic fuel. Triglyceride fatty acids (TGFA) are primarily stored. Fetal glucose needs are minimal at this stage. In late gestation, free fatty acids (FFA) and triglyceride fatty acids (TGFA) are seen as the primary maternal metabolic fuels and glucose is diverted from maternal tissues for placental–fetal transport.

Table 5   Effect of Calorie Restriction in a Third Trimester Pregnant Diabetic: H. H.[a]

	Study Days				
	1	5	7	13	20
Diet (kcal)	1200	2000	2000	2000	2000
Weight (kg)	83.4	83.6	84.0	—	87.6
Insulin (units)	50	50	55	55	55
Plasma					
Glucose (mg/dl)	114	119	101	92	115
FFA (μEq/L)	465	485	420	390	235
TG (mg/dl)	354	384	347	311	254
Urinary					
Glucose	0	0	0	0	0
Ketones	Lge	Neg	Neg	Neg	Neg

[a] FFA = free fatty acids; TG = triglyceride; Lge = large.

EFFECTS OF EXPERIMENTAL DIETS IN NORMAL AND DIABETIC PREGNANCY

Recently, it has been found that feeding a high carbohydrate diet to adult-onset diabetics can decrease fasting glucose, improve glucose tolerance, and reduce fasting insulin (34). A transient rise in fasting triglycerides is also observed (34). Since pregnancy is characterized by a two- to threefold increase in fasting triglycerides in late gestation (Table 4) (35), we anticipated that hypertriglyceridemia in pregnancy would be exaggerated by "carbohydrate induction," with corresponding declines in fasting glucose and insulin (36).

Results of a 40% carbohydrate diet for 3 days and a 75% carbohydrate diet for 5 to 7 days in pregnancy are presented in Figure 6. Four subjects were studied in the third trimester, and two postpartum. Subject K was a mild diabetic treated with 15 to 30 units of insulin, subject B was a gestational diabetic not treated with insulin, and subjects G and R were normal. For subject K, the triglyceride response was lowest in the third trimester and greatest during lactation. The three other subjects showed similarly modest responses in total and VLDL triglycerides in the third trimester. By contrast, the two postpartum nonlactating studies showed a greater triglyceride response in both absolute and relative terms. For instance, VLDL triglyceride increased

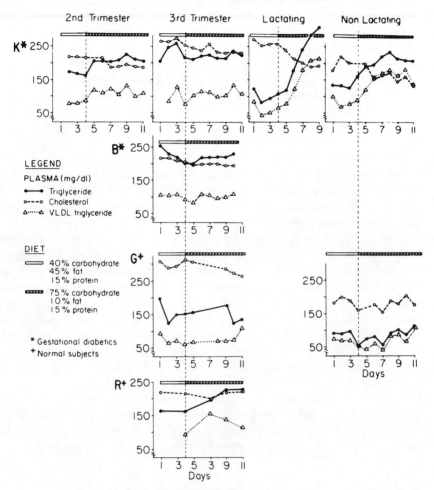

**EFFECT OF HIGH CARBOHYDRATE FEEDING
ON PLASMA LIPIDS IN PREGNANCY**

Figure 6. Total plasma and VLDL triglyceride and total plasma cholesterol are shown in four pregnant subjects fed baseline diet for 3 days and high carbohydrate diet for 5 to 7 days. Subjects K and B were studied on a metabolic ward; G and R were studied at home. Diets consisted of measured amounts of a mixed diet. Subjects K and B were mild diabetics, with subject K receiving 15 units of insulin in the second trimester and 30 units in the third trimester. Subjects G and R had normal glucose tolerance. Reprinted by permission of publishers.

131

$17 \pm 6\%$ (mean $\pm$ SD) in the four third trimester subjects compared to a $68 \pm 19\%$ increment in the two postpartum nonlactating studies ($p <$ 0.025). The conclusion from these observations is that the control of hypertriglyceridemia in human pregnancy differs from other hyper-triglyceridemias, where high carbohydrate feeding exaggerates the hypertriglyceridemia (see (36) for a further discussion of this question). Whatever the mechanism, maternal triglyceride homeostasis appears to be maintained in a narrow range independent of diet, possibly to meet a continuing need for triglyceride fatty acids by mother or fetus.

The effects of diet on plasma glucose, FFA, and insulin are shown in Table 6. On high carbohydrate feeding, fasting glucose levels did not worsen in the two diabetics, K and B, and may have improved in sub-ject K, particularly postpartum. Similarly, fasting FFA levels declined slightly on high carbohydrate feeding both antepartum and postpartum. Plasma insulin in the three subjects in whom it could be measured was not consistently altered by high carbohydrate feeding. Evaluation is needed of the glycemic response to high carbohydrate feeding during the day in the pregnant diabetic.

The effect of diets of differing composition on the rat pregnancy model are being evaluated in ongoing studies by Dr. Marian Childs in our laboratory (Table 7). Over a 9-day period from day 12 to day 21 of gestation, pregnant rats consumed more calories on the nonfat sucrose and on 15% fat diets than on the nonfat starch diets, to which they adapted rather slowly. While maternal weight gain was less in the starch fed rats, the efficiency of caloric utilization was the same in all four groups of rats. While the mother was perhaps able to utilize the calories provided, the pups of sucrose fed mothers were significantly lighter than those of the fat fed mothers, and nonsignificantly lighter ($p < 0.1$) than those of the starch fed mothers. Since essential fatty acids were provided in both high carbohydrate diets, the decreased weight of the sucrose fed pups indicates that the quality of the calories as well as the quantity of calories of the maternal diet can affect fetal growth.

CALORIE INTAKE IN DIABETIC PREGNANCY

From the foregoing review, it should be possible to arrive at a sensible and practical program for dietary management of the pregnant diabetic. The first point to remember is that diabetic diets for nonpregnant persons take two major forms: a calorie restricted carbohydrate con-trolled diet in the obese adult-onset, ketosis-resistant diabetic, and a weight maintaining diet with careful allocation of dietary carbohydrate

Table 6   Mean Fasting Plasma Glucose and FFA during Baseline and High Carbohydrate Diets in Pregnancy and Postpartum

Plasma	Subject	Pregnancy		Postpartum	
		B	H	B	H
Glucose (mg/dl)	K	104 ± 6^a	94 ± 10	111 ± 2	101 ± 6^b
	B	88 ± 8	90 ± 7	—	
	G	66 ± 5	64 ± 2	69 ± 1	70 ± 2
	R	73 ± 8	72 ± 6	—	—
FFA (Eq/L)	K	629 ± 67	632 ± 49	818 ± 50	854 ± 109
	B	623 ± 113	588 ± 47	—	—
	G	990 ± 148	788 ± 50	880 ± 118	616 ± 142^c
	R	1223 ± 146	1053 ± 160	—	—
IRI (U/ml)	K^d	—	—	—	—
	B	27 ± 18	27 ± 11	—	—
	G	9 ± 7	12 ± 5	16 ± 4	8 ± 13
	R	15 ± 1	12 ± 2	—	—

[a] Mean $\pm$ SD of 3 baseline days and 5 to 7 high carbohydrate feeding days.
[b] Significant differences between B (baseline) and H (high carbohydrate): $p <$ 0.005.
[c] Significant differences between B and H: $p < 0.025$.
[d] IRI not measured in subject K because of antibody interference in this insulin treated subject; B is a gestational diabetic, G and R are normal.

throughout the day to minimize swings in glycemia (1) in the juvenile, ketosis prone diabetic.

How do these principles apply to the pregnant diabetic? In general, the stable, overweight, "adult-onset" diabetic mother in pregnancy will fall into the category of White class A or the White class B diabetic. It is in these groups in particular that the question is raised whether calorie restriction should be employed as part of the diabetic treatment during pregnancy (Table 8). In general, the White class C–F pregnant diabetics will be labile and ketosis prone, have normal body weight, and have an obligatory requirement for insulin and a normal calorie increment in pregnancy (Table 8).

Since ketonuria and ketosis occur much more rapidly on fasting in the pregnant mother and even more rapidly in the pregnant diabetic, and since ketonuria is associated directly or indirectly with injury to central nervous system development of the baby, calorie restriction cannot be

Table 7   Effects of Changes in Diet Composition on Weight Gain Between Days 9 and 21 in Rat Gestation

	Starch	Sucrose	Fat
% Composition (by calories)			
Carbohydrate	75.2	75.2	47.2
Fat	0.8	0.8	33
Protein	24	24	20
Mean daily			
Intake (kcal)	58 ± 4[a]	91 ± 4[b]	78 ± 6[b]
Weight gain (g)	7.4 ± 1.0	11.2 ± 0.4[b]	10.4 ± 0.5[b]
Weight gain (g/100 kcal)	12.8 ± 0.1	12.4 ± 0.7	13.4 ± 0.6
Fetus weight (g)	3.6 ± 0.1	3.3 ± 0.1	3.6 ± 0.03[c]

[a] Mean ± SEM.
[b] Significantly different from starch ($p < 0.05$).
[c] Significantly different from sucrose ($p < 0.02$).

advocated as the prime therapy of the obese pregnant diabetic. The prime deficiency to be treated is the lack of insulin effectiveness, which must be treated with insulin replacement. Finally, in one pregnancy that we have observed, food restriction to the point of ketonuria did not accomplish glycemic control.

While food restriction to the extent of negative caloric balance is not advisable for any pregnant woman, there may be a place for limiting food intake in the mother inclined to eat beyond the calorie increment considered appropriate to normal pregnancy. A number of points must be considered with this therapeutic course (Table 9). A calorie increment sufficient to produce appropriate weight gain must be selected. This weight gain may vary from approximately 27.5 lb at term in a normal weight mother down to 19 lb at term in an obese mother (12,37). Serial weight measurement must be accurate and approximately no less than 1 lb/wk in the normal mother, and 0.7 lb/wk in the obese mother. Weight gain as fat (primarily a second trimester event) must not be confused with weight gain as edema, hydramnios, or an overweight baby and placenta. A careful nutritional history must be obtained before intervention to ensure that important nutrients are not arbitrarily eliminated, particularly if the diet is of poor quality. Also the caloric prescription must take into account the mother's activity level. Finally, urinary ketones should be monitored to be sure that the calorie "control" has not become excessive.

Since obese mothers tend to gain less weight and lean mothers more weight in pregnancy (Table 3) (12,37), Hytten suggests that there is a "leveling effect" of pregnancy on body fatness. It may be that the insensitive satiety center of the obese person is activated in pregnancy (12). While it is not known if this mechanism operates in the obese pregnant diabetic, the difficulty of accurately measuring weekly weight gain and supervising caloric intake makes reliance on the mother's appetite center highly attractive. In short, the instances where the mother's food intake must be seriously restricted should be relatively few.

Recognition of the undesirability of negative caloric balance in diabetic pregnancy requires that greater reliance be placed on insulin therapy in the treatment of the mother's diabetes. An application of this concept is insulin therapy of the gestational diabetic which is of proved value in reducing the morbidity of excess fetal adiposity (38) and possibly the mortality as well (39).

DIET COMPOSITION

Based on our dietary observations in human pregnancy, diabetic control appears to be little affected by the high carbohydrate diet. Our results are in accord with more extensive studies of high carbohydrate diet in nonpregnant diabetics, where diabetic control over the 24-hour period does not appear to be affected (40). In other words, there appears to be no more reason to restrict carbohydrate in diabetic pregnancy than in other diabetics. Some dietary fat is advisable, since it tends to delay gastric emptying, but fat increases above 45% as calories should be avoided at least on theoretical grounds to prevent diet-induced ketogenesis. Administration of dietary carbohydrate in a form associated

Table 8   Therapy of Diabetes Mellitus

Adult onset			
Weight reduction	A	±	? weight
± Insulin	B	+	reduction
Juvenile onset	C	+	
Obligate insulin Rx	D	+	
Spacing carb. calories	F	+	Spacing
Consistency in timing and			of carb.
amounts of food eaten	R	+	calories

Table 9   Questions in Treating Excess Maternal Weight Gain

1. How to define excess gain?
2. How to measure excess gain?
3. How to distinguish excess gain from:
   hydramnios?
   edema?
   overweight fetus and placenta?
4. How to guard against nutritional deprivation?
5. How to determine what foods to restrict?

with natural fiber appears desirable in light of recent reports that guar gum can reduce the rate of glucose absorption from the gut (41) and the degree of glycosuria (42). Which forms of carbohydrates have the greatest hyperglycemic effect is still under study (43). Until this question is resolved, refined concentrated sugars should be avoided in the diet of the pregnant diabetic.

DISTRIBUTION OF DIETARY CARBOHYDRATE

As pointed out by West (1), the amount and spacing of dietary carbohydrate is crucial in the diet of the insulin-dependent, labile diabetic. As insulin has increased importance relative to calorie restriction in diabetic pregnancy, the timing and amount of the daily carbohydrate intake also takes on increased importance.

Because of the likelihood that insulin is degraded more rapidly by placental enzymes in late gestation (44), mixtures of short and intermediate acting insulins are often administered morning and evening beginning in midgestation in the labile diabetic and in the third trimester in the stable diabetic. With the varied insulin regimens, the typical times for insulin reaction may change, requiring changes in the timing and amounts of carbohydrate feeding. While no rigid rules can be set down, the principle cannot be overstated that diet serves as handmaiden to insulin therapy in the diabetic pregnancy to minimize peaks and valleys of the glycemic changes throughout the day. Successful application of this principle requires not only a clinician, a dietician, and a patient able to implement the necessary dietary measures, but also sufficient blood glucose monitoring information upon which to make recommendations about insulin and the diet. Blood glucose monitoring is necessary since urinary glycosuria is often erratic or absent with a reasonable degree of glycemic control in diabetic pregnancy. Examples of hospital blood glucose monitoring have been reported (45,46), but outpatient monitoring schemes can also be devised using local clinical labs or detrostix monitoring.

SUMMARY

The tendency of the pregnant diabetic to fasting ketosis limits the extent to which calorie restriction (particularly negative caloric balance) can be used in the treatment of the obese, adult-onset, pregnant diabetic. In addition, the vagaries of measuring excess weight gain and detecting extraneous sources of weight gain in diabetic pregnancy, and the difficulty of accurately enforcing a caloric prescription without forcing the subject to weigh her food, make the determination of an accurate degree of calorie limitation difficult at best. A greater reliance on the mother's appetite center may be more accurate and rewarding in most instances than any devices available to the clinician.

Important considerations in the diet of the pregnant diabetic are adequate protein, minerals, and vitamins, an amount of carbohydrate that is constant from day to day but not necessarily restricted, carbohydrate intake in an unrefined form that maximizes the intake of associated fiber, and a reproducible meal and snack schedule which complements the insulin regimen. Insulin must remain the primary therapeutic tool if the effects of maternal diabetes on fetal morbidity and mortality are to be minimized.

ACKNOWLEDGMENTS

The authors are grateful to Linda Lillard and Nikki Silver for secretarial assistance and to Kathy Stamm who reviewed the manuscript. This work has been supported in part by grant HD-AM-08968 and contract NO1-HV-2157-L.

REFERENCES

1. K. M. West, *Ann. Int. Med.,* **79,** 425 (1973).

2. F. C. Wood and E. L. Bierman, *Nutr. Today,* **7,** 4 (1972).

3. R. M. Pitkin, in J. E. Tyson, Ed., *Symposium on Pregnancy, Med. Clin. N.A.,* **61,** 3 (1977).

4. Committee on Maternal Nutrition, Food and Nutrition Board, *Maternal Nutrition and the Course of Pregnancy, Summary Report,* National Academy of Sciences, Wash. D.C., 1970, pp. 1–23.

5. F. E. Hytten and I. Leitch, *The Physiology of Human Pregnancy,* 2nd ed., *Blackwell,* Oxford, 1971, pp. 333–439.

6. P. White, in A. Marble, P. White, R. F. Bradley, and L. F. Krall, Eds., *Joslin's Diabetes Mellitus,* 11th Ed., Lea and Febiger, Philadelphia, 1971, pp. 581–98.

7. J. Pedersen, in R. A. Camerini-Davalos and H. S. Cole, Eds., *Early Diabetes in Early Life,* Academic, New York, 1975, pp. 381–91.

8. D. Younger, in K. E. Sussman and R. J. S. Metz, *Diabetes Mellitus,* 4th Ed., Amer. Diabetes Assoc., New York, 1975, pp. 135–45.

9. R. W. Beard and N. W. Oakley, in R. W. Beard and P. W. Nathanielsz, London, 1976, pp. 137–57.

10. R. DeHertogh, *Louvain Med., 96,* 139 (1977).

11. P. Felig, in J. E. Tyson, Ed., *Symposium on Pregnancy, Med. Clin. N.A., 61,* 43 (1977).

12. F. E. Hytten, A. M. Thomson, and N. Taggart, *J. Obstet. Gynaecol. Br. Commonw., 73,* 553 (1966).

13. G. H. Beaton, J. Beare, M. H. Ryu, and E. W. McHenry, *J. Nutr., 54,* 291 (1954).

14. J. Seitchik, *Obstet. Gynecol., 29,* 155 (1967).

15. K. Emerson, E. L. Poindexter, and M. Kothari, *Obstet. Gynecol., 45,* 505 (1975).

16. L. J. Poo, W. Lew, and T. Addis, *J. Biol. Chem., 128,* 69 (1939).

17. K. Emerson, B. N. Saxena, and E. L. Poindexter, *Obstet. Gynecol., 40,* 786 (1972).

18. R. H. Knopp, C. D. Saudek, R. A. Arky, and J. B. O'Sullivan, *Endocrinology, 92,* 984 (1973).

19a. R. H. Knopp, A. Montes and M. R. Warth, in *Laboratory Indices of Nutritional Pregnancy,* National Acad. Sci, (U.S.A.), Wash. D.C. (in press) 1978.

19b. R. H. Knopp, *Contemp. Ob. Gyn.* (in press) (1978).

20. R. H. Knopp, H. J. Ruder, E. Herrera, and N. Freinkel, *Acta Endocrinol., 65,* 352 (1970).

21. M. M. Grumbach, S. L. Kaplan, J. J. Sciarra, and I. M. Burr, *Ann. N.Y. Acad. Sci., 148,* 501 (1965).

22. M. Talaat, Y. A. Habib, and A. M. Higazy, *Arch. Int. Pharmacodyn. Ther., 154,* 402 (1965).

23. R. K. Kalkhoff, M. Jacobson, and D. Lemper, *J. Clin. Endocrinol. Metab., 31,* 24 (1970).

24. N. Freinkel, in G. S. Liebel and G. A. Wrenshall, Eds., *On the Nature and Treatment of Diabetes,* Excerpta Medica Foundation, Amsterdam, 1965, pp. 679–91.

25. B. Persson and N. O. Lunell, *Am. J. Obstet. Gynecol., 122,* 737 (1975).

26. E. Herrera, R. H. Knopp, and N. Freinkel, *J. Clin. Invest., 48,* 2260 (1969).

27. P. Felig and V. Lynch, *Science, 170,* 990 (1970).

28. J. Pedersen, *The Pregnant Diabetic and Her Newborn*, Williams and Wilkins, Baltimore, 1967, pp. 32–34.

29. K. Emerson, B. N. Saxena, S. K. Varma, and E. L. Poindexter, *Obstet. Gynecol.*, **43**, 354 (1974).

30. J. A. Churchill and H. W. Berendes, *Am. J. Obstet. Gynecol.*, **105**, 257 (1969).

31. J. A. Churchill and H. W. Berendes, in *Perinatal Factors Affecting Human Development*, Scientific Publication #185, Wash. D.C., Pan American Health Organization, 1969.

32. H. W. Berendes, in R. A. Camerini-Davalos and H. S. Cole, Eds., *Early Diabetes in Early Life*, Academic, New York, 1975, pp. 135–40.

33. G. A. Stehbens, G. L. Baker, and M. Kitchell, *Obstet. Gynecol.*, **127**, 408 (1977).

34. J. D. Brunzell, R. L. Lerner, W. R. Hazzard, D. Porte, Jr., and E. L. Bierman, *New Engl. J. Med.*, **284**, 521 (1971).

35. M. R. Warth and R. H. Knopp, *J. Clin. Endocrinol. Metab.*, **41**, 649 (1975).

36. M. R. Warth and R. H. Knopp, *Diabetes* (in press).

37. C. H. Peckham and R. E. Christianson, *Am. J. Obstet. Gynecol.*, **111**, 1 (1971).

38. J. B. O'Sullivan, S. S. Gellis, R. V. Dandrow, and B. O. Tenney, *Obstet. Gynecol.*, **27**, 683 (1966).

39. J. B. O'Sullivan, In R. A. Camerini-Davalos and H. S. Cole, Eds., *Early Diabetes in Early Life*, Academic, N.Y., 1975, pp. 447–53.

40. T. G. Kiehm, J.W. Anderson, and K. Ward, *Am. J. Clin. Nutr.*, **29**, 895 (1976).

41. D. J. A. Jenkins, D. V. Goff, A. R. Leeds, K. G. M. M. Alberti, T. M. S. Wolever, M. A. Gassull, and T. D. R. Hockaday, *Lancet*, **2**, 172 (1976).

42. D. J. A. Jenkins, T. D. R. Hockaday, R. Howart, E. C. Apling, T. M. S. Wolever, A. R. Leeds, S. Bacon, and J. Dilawari, *Lancet*, **2**, 779 (1977).

43. R. A. Lenner, *Am. J., Clin. Nutr.*, **29**, 716 (1976).

44. N. Freinkel and C. J. Goodner, *J. Clin. Invest.*, **39**, 116 (1960).

45. M. D. G. Gillmer, R. W. Beard, F. M. Brooke, and N. W. Oakley, *Brit. Med. J.*, **3**, 399 (1975).

46. S. B. Lewis, W. K. Murray, J. D. Wallin, D. R. Coustan, T. A. Daane, D. R. Treadway, and J. P. Navins, *Obstet. Gynecol.*, **48**, 260 (1976).

PART 5

Lipids

10

Genetic Obesity
in Man and Rodents

M. R. C. GREENWOOD and M. P. CLEARY

Institute of Human Nutrition and Department of Human Genetics and Development,
College of Physicians and Surgeons, Columbia University, New York, New York

and

JULES HIRSCH

The Rockefeller University, New York, New York

It is well known that obesity tends to occur in humans among kindreds, and that its incidence is greater in some socioeconomic and ethnic groups than in others (1). However, it has thus far been impossible to define clearly the contributions of nature, that is, inheritability, from those of nurture.

Population statistics on the prevalence of overweight and obesity have been particularly difficult to evaluate. The evaluation of the results is dependent upon the criteria used to define overweight and obesity and the characteristics of the population under consideration, such as age, sex, ethnic group, and socioeconomic status (2-4). Therefore, statistics will not be discussed here in great detail. However, examples do bear

Supported in part by NIH Grants HD 08965/12637; HD 07000 and AM 18325, and grants from the Nutrition Foundation and National Foundation–March of Dimes. A portion of the material included in the first section of this chapter comprised a part of the Ph.D. dissertation submitted to Columbia University by M. P. Cleary. M. R. C. Greenwood's present address and title: Associate Professor of Biology, Vassar College, Poughkeepsie, New York. M. P. Cleary's present address and title: Assistant Professor, Department of Nutrition and Food Sciences, Drexel University, Philadelphia, Pennsylvania.

noting to establish that obesity does affect a large number of Americans. A recent report from a United States Senate committee stated that overweight and obesity afflict close to 30% of Americans (5). Obesity in infants is not well documented in the United States, but in a recent study on a group of 300 normal British infants under 1 year of age, the overall rate of overweight (110 to 120% of standard weight) was 44% (6). The prevalence of overweight in a group of preschool children in Manhattan was found to be 13% (7). An evaluation of weights in children in primary and secondary schools in several Boston suburbs revealed that overweight and obesity occurred in 10 to 16% (8). An increase in the prevalence of obesity and overweight has been seen throughout the adult years in the American population (9).

The cause, or causes, of this apparent epidemic of excess poundage is not known. Various explanations have been put forth, based on changes in the environment such as increases in refined carbohydrate consumption (10), decreases in breastfeeding and earlier weaning of infants (6,11,12), and decreases in energy expenditure with no decrease in caloric intake (13,14). In particular, infant feeding has changed in the twentieth century. Infants who were once breast-fed through the first year of life are now being fed artificial formulas which are frequently supplemented with solid food as early as the first or second week of life (12,15). Increased body weights of infants have been shown to correspond to daily food intakes in excess of those recommended (15). It has been reported that breast-fed babies usually have solid food added to their diets at a much later age and do not double their birth weights as quickly as bottle-fed babies (16).

FAMILIAL TRENDS IN OBESITY

The importance of hereditary factors in producing obesity in humans is not clear. Animal studies have clearly shown that obesity can be inherited (see later sections), and some human studies have also demonstrated a familial pattern in obesity (17,18). Mossberg, in a study of 504 obese children, noted that obese children more frequently had obese parents than did nonobese children (19). Mayer has reviewed the available information on the incidence of obesity in offspring from various types of matings. Two obese parents have a 73% chance of having an obese child; one obese and one normal parent, a 33% chance; and two normal parents, a 9% chance. A recent analysis of data accumulated from the Ten State Nutrition Survey has also shown strong familial correlations of fatness (17). For example, by age 17, children who had two obese parents were three times fatter (assessed by fatfold, or skinfold thickness) than children of two lean parents. The importance of environment in determining such statistics on the general population is pointed out by similar results reported in this same population for adopted and foster children (20,21).

Genetic factors may be more clearly indicated in studies of twins. Comparisons of body weights in monozygotic twins, dizygotic twins, and like-sexed siblings have indicated that the strongest correlation occurs in identical twins, regardless of whether they are raised in the same environment (22–24). A recent study of 101 twin pairs, with at least one twin being overweight, strongly suggests that genetic factors play a role in the development of some human obesities (25). As shown in Table 1, monozygotic twin pairs had much smaller intrapair difference for skinfold thickness at these different sites than dizygotic twin pairs. A similar twin study by Brook et al., which divided the pairs into older and younger age groups, concluded that environment affected body fatness to a greater extent in the younger children (26). However, in the older age group the genetic influence appeared to override the earlier environmental effects.

Although theories, such as the glucostatic theory and the lipostatic theory, have been proposed in attempts to explain short term satiety and long term body weight regulation, there is no consensus about what the critical lesion or lesions are that result in the pathology leading to obesity. It seems likely that obesity is a pathology of multiple causes. Since the primary site of the excess storage of fat is adipose tissue, an understanding of the development of adipose tissue is necessary in order

Table 1   Comparison between Monozygotic and Dizygotic Twin Pairs—Intrapair Differences of Skinfold Measurement[a]

Twin Type	Location of Skinfold Measurement	No. of Pairs	Intrapair Difference $\times$ (1/10 mm)
MZ	Triceps	40	23
DZ	Triceps	61	75
MZ	Subscapular	40	40
DZ	Subscapular	61	133
MZ	Abdominal	38	34
DZ	Abdominal	60	99

[a] Adapted from Borjeson (25).

to unravel the dysfunctions leading to obesity. When normal adipose tissue development is more clearly understood, it will be easier to detect changes that may be involved in the etiology or maintenance of obesity.

THE DEVELOPMENT OF OBESITY IN HUMANS

As with many biomedical research problems, investigation into the development of human fat resulted from an awareness of obesity as an increasing public health concern. Early studies of adipose tissue development were mainly concerned with manifest obesity and attempts to treat overweight individuals. From these studies some interesting observations were made which have helped to clarify some of the problems that arise when studying adipose tissue.

A particularly interesting study was published in the late 1950s by Mullins on overweight adults being treated for weight reduction (29). Over 100 obese adults were interviewed and it was discovered that one-third of them reported being obese as children (29). These tended to be the more severely obese. Severity was defined by Mullins in terms of percent overweight as mild (20 to 25% overweight), moderate (25 to 50% overweight), and severe (more than 50% overweight). Of the subjects reporting a history of juvenile-onset obesity 53% were more than 50% overweight, whereas only 29% of the adult-onset obese individuals fell into this category (Table 2). In addition, those reporting juvenile obesity also reported obesity more frequently in near relatives. There was a higher incidence of failure following treatment in the juvenile-onset obese group.

Over the past decade considerably more data have accrued from several laboratories (30–33), suggesting that human obesity may have distinct subgroups which can be classified by adipose tissue morphology. The two major types of human obesity, hypertrophic and hyperplastic-

Table 2 Severity of Obesity in Obese Adults in Relation to Age of Onset of Obesity[a]

	Mild Obesity	Moderate Obesity	Severe Obesity
Childhood-onset obesity	12%	35%	53%
Adult-onset obesity	41%	30%	29%

[a] From Mullins (29).

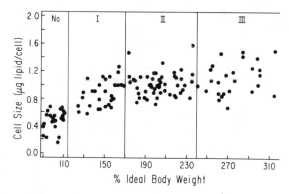

Figure 1.   Cell size of adults related to percent of ideal body weight (32).

hypertrophic, are the most common, but a few cases of purely hyperplastic obesity have also been reported. The earliest analysis of the data
suggested a strong correlation between early age of onset of obesity and
the hyperplastic-hypertrophic form of obesity. This correlation continues
to be true and, as we shall discuss later, very obese preschool children are
commonly of the hyperplastic-hypertrophic type. However, as more
obese individuals are studied it has become clear that certain types of individuals who become very obese may become hyperplastic even when they
have no history of childhood obesity.

For example, when a group of 106 obese and 32 normal patients
were examined for alterations in adipose tissue morphology several
consistent relationships emerged (32). Figure 1 shows that even with
moderate degrees of obesity there is already an increase in fat cell size
compared to nonobese. Within the nonobese group there is a good deal
of variance in fat cell size but no evidence that a slightly chubbier or
slightly less chubby individual has a difference in cell size in this group.
With greater degrees of obesity fat cell size does not continue to increase
markedly. Therefore, hypertrophy is a marker of obesity; as nearly
every obese individual has a bigger fat cell, but increased fat cell size
does not correlate with the degree of obesity.

Figure 2 shows fat cell number in the same individuals. It is apparent
that with small degrees of obesity fat cell number does not change at all.
However, as obesity becomes more and more marked, fat cell number
increases according to the degree of obesity.

Figure 3 summarizes the fat cell size and number data. These data
indicate the proportional effects of degrees of obesity on fat cell size and
cell number. Fat cell size changes even with the most minimal degree of
obesity and remains more or less the same across various degrees of

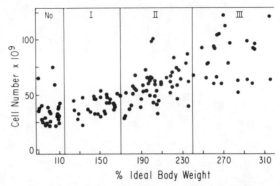

Figure 2.   Cell number of adults related to percent of ideal body weight (32).

obesity, whereas fat cell number is hardly changed by a mild amount of obesity but is markedly changed as obesity becomes more severe.

If one plots cell size versus cell number (Fig. 3), it is evident that those who are most severely obese, who would have the greatest product of cell size times cell number, are those who are most hyperplastic, that is, they have the largest number of cells as well, which may suggest that at least some humans, like some rat strains, may produce new fat cells in response to severe hypertrophy even in adulthood. Whether this "susceptibility" is at all inherited is most interesting and as yet unknown.

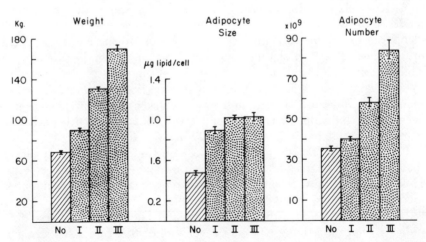

Figure 3.   Summary of cellularity data for all obese adults compared to nonobese adults (32).

The success rate of weight loss for adult dieters is quite variable, depending on type of treatment, degree of overweight, age of onset of obesity, and length of follow-up study (29, 34–36). Additionally, individuals with a long history of obesity have even greater difficulties in maintaining weight losses. This may be related to the fact that weight loss produces decreases in fat cell size with no change in fat cell number (30,31,37). Nevertheless, for whatever reason, those individuals whose obesity is characterized by increases both in the number as well as in the size of fat cells are definitely at a disadvantage with respect to "curing" their obesity and show high rates of recidivism.

CHILDHOOD OBESITY

The fact that obese adults, particularly those with hyperplastic childhood-onset obesity, are more severely affected and do not maintain weight loss makes it imperative to turn attention to the normal and abnormal development of adipose tissue in children. Currently available methodologies have indicated that normal adipose tissue cellularity develops in humans by proceeding through several stages. In infants fat cell number tripled or quadrupled to approximately 10×10^9 from birth to 2 years of age (30). During this same time fat cell size also increased. Fat cell number in normal children did not appear to change in any significantly observable degree from 2 to 10 years of age (38–40). Adult fat cell number in a range from 25 to 40×10^9 cells was attained at some point after puberty (38,39,41). Fat cell size remained constant from 2 to 12 years, reaching adult values at some later time (30,40,41). Skinfold measurements, which are frequently used to indicate the quantity of total body fatness, have been shown to parallel the changes seen in fat cell size and number (42). Although the critical period for prenatal fat cell number development is unknown, the third trimester of gestation has been thought to be the most likely period (38,43,44).

Many studies of the abnormal fat accumulation in obese children have offered promising insights into the developmental aspects of obesity. Obese children over the age of 2 who were more than 130% of ideal body weight were found to have enlarged fat cell size compared to fat cell size of normal weight children (7,45,46). Fat cell number of the obese children exceeded that of normal children and frequently exceeded normal adult values. Furthermore, Knittle et al. have reported that fat cell number in obese children increases at ages when normal weight children showed no changes in fat cell number (46) (Fig. 4). This indi-

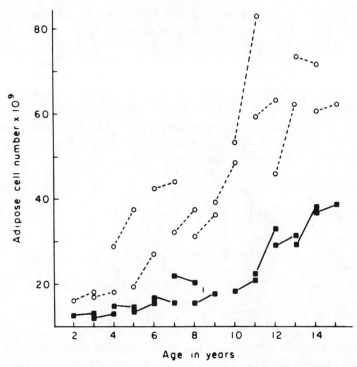

Figure 4. Adipose cell number of obese children (0----0) and normal children (■————■) (46).

cates that obese children display a change in the development of fat cell size and number.

In another group of 54 obese children ranging in age from 0.8 to 16.6 years, whose weight exceeded the expected for height by at least 20% and whose triceps and subscapular skinfold thicknesses were over the 90th percentile, two different patterns of adipose cellularity were apparent (38,39). An early-onset obesity, which had been evident by 1 year of age, was found in 29 of the 54 obese children. The remaining 25 obese children had become obese later in childhood and were classified as late onset. Both groups of children were grossly overweight, with similar percents of body weight as fat (see Table 3). Early-onset obese children had significantly smaller fat cell size than late-onset obese children, while both groups had significantly larger fat cell size than control children (Table 3). In addition, the two groups of obese children had very different fat cell numbers. Sixty percent of the early-onset children had a fat cell number that was two standard deviations above

Table 3   Percent Overweight, Percent Body Weight as Fat, and Adipose Cell Size in Obese and Normal Children[a,b]

	% Overweight	% Body Weight as Fat	Adipose Cell Size (μg Lipid/Cell
Control	—	17.5	0.30
Early-onset obese	52.3	38.2	0.64
Late-onset obese	52.7	36.7	0.77

[a] From Brook (39).
[b] Cells from obese children contained more lipid than controls ($p < 0.001$). Cells from early-onset obese children contained less lipid than from late-onset obese ($p < 0.01$).

the mean for normal children matched for age, while only 4% of the late-onset children had a fat cell number in this range (Fig. 5). Skeletal maturity was advanced in the early-onset group of children but not in the late-onset group. Even when the fat cell number in the former group was corrected for this factor, it remained significantly greater than that of late-onset obese or normal children.

Forbes (47) has identified two groups of obese children, "the first characterized by a definite increase in LBM (lean body mass) as well as

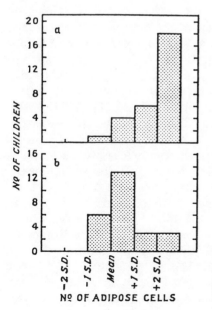

Figure 5. Cellularity of obese children compared to normal children. (a) Fat cell number in early-onset obesity. (b) Fat cell number in late-onset obesity (38).

fat, the second in which excess body weight is due exclusively to the accumulation of fat." The group with increased LBM also had more advanced bone age and a history of obesity since infancy. The other group was usually of normal height and had become obese in middle or late childhood. Cheek and co-workers also studied body composition of obese adolescents (48). Two different groups were identified with respect to bone age, muscle development, and fat, but there was no clear-cut correlation with age of onset of obesity. These data were difficult to compare to Forbes' because not all of Cheek's subjects were tested for all variables within that particular study nor were the same variables examined in both studies.

These studies have pointed out that hyperplastic obesity can indeed be seen in childhood and is evident at an early age. Children as young as 2 years of age have been noted to have fat cell number in the adult range (39,40). In addition, the data suggest that there are possibly two types of obesities identifiable during childhood, but do not clarify to what extent these types are genetically determined.

An important question is whether intervention during the childhood years could alter the course of the accumulation of lipid-filled fat cells. If the factors contributing to fat cell hypertrophy and hyperplasia were primarily environmental, it would follow that changing the environment should alter the course of the developing obesity. Theoretically, since the accumulation of fat cells is still in progress during early childhood, intervention could possibly prevent further accretion of cells. Nonetheless, most studies of children treated for obesity have not been encouraging. Lloyd et al. reexamined 98 children 9 years after initial weight loss as a result of dietary treatment (49). At the time of intervention the children ranged in age from 1 to 14 years and were given 1000 kcal/ day, which included 50 to 60 g of protein (50). Amphetamine sulfate was given as an appetite suppressant. Final heights of the children who had gone through puberty were significantly below the expected. Despite previous weight losses, 80% of the subjects were grossly overweight at follow-up. Even the group of children whose weight loss had brought them close to normal levels did not differ in weight at follow-up from those who had responded poorly to treatment.

In a combined program of diet, appetite suppressants, and physical activity, 77% of 122 obese children were still obese 2 to 8 years after therapy (51). One to five years after similar therapy, 82% of another group of children initially above the 90th percentile for body weight remained overweight when reevaluated (52).

Recent work by Knittle and Ginsberg-Fellner offers some slight encouragement in the treatment of obese children (7). Obese children with hypercellular fat depots, between the ages of 2 to 11 years, were treated in the hospital with a diet of 400 kcal/day plus iron and vitamin supplementation. Weight loss resulted in decreased fat cell size with no decrease in fat cell number. Maintenance of weight loss and cessation of further increases in fat cell number appeared possible using this approach when the initial total fat cell number was below the lower adult range of from 25 to 35 $\times$ 10^9 cells. However, it will be necessary to follow these children through adolescence and into adulthood to evaluate the permanent effects of this form of treatment.

An evaluation of the data presented thus far indicates that obesity which had manifested itself in childhood and was maintained into adulthood was accompanied by increased fat cell number, that is, hyperplasia of fat depots. Hyperplasia has been found in childhood and was most severe in the cases of earliest onset. Dietary intervention in the child or adult can result in weight loss, but maintenance of a normal body weight has been difficult and has usually not been achieved. In addition, fat cell number does not decrease with weight loss and it is unknown at this time if prevention of further increases by dietary intervention in the preschool obese child can be maintained until adulthood. Therefore, it would appear that a means of predicting childhood obesity before it severely manifests itself would be desirable. That is, some means of recognizing the individual at risk for increased body fat if present dietary practices are continued would be helpful in determining the need for intervention.

DETECTION OF HUMAN OBESITY

Various attempts at early identification have been undertaken. Birth weights have been examined retrospectively and prospectively, but in most cases do not appear to be reliable indicators of later obesity (15,53–55). In fact, one investigator has even suggested that low birth weight may make a child more susceptible to rapid postnatal weight gain and later obesity (56). Presumably obesity in low birth weight infants could result from excessive catch-up growth (15,57).

A cross-sectional study of 300 infants under the age of 1 year in Dudley, Worcestershire, showed that although many infants appear by weight to be obese (120% greater than standard weight) or overweight (110 to 120% greater than standard weight) at either 3 (47.7%) or 6 (54.6%) months after birth, the rate had dropped to 27.4% by 1 year of age (6). Obesity decreased by 75% between 6 months and 12 months of age. It is difficult to draw conclusions from these data since individual babies were not reassessed to see if they continued to follow this pattern. These results suggest that perhaps there is a normally high rate of apparent obesity and overweight in young infants as a consequence of current feeding practices which corrects itself as babies become able to respond to satiety signals that may not be fully developed in the young infant (58). It has also been suggested that infants increase their activity levels at 6 months and the percentage of body fat normally decreases (Widdowson, 1974).

Since birth weight is not a good predictor, rapid weight gain in the first 6 months of life has been suggested as an indicator of obesity in infants (56,59). Crawford assessed 13 anthropomorphic measurements including birth weights and lengths of 448 infants between 25 and 29 weeks of age (59). An additional nine variables were computed from the primary measurements. Weight gain from birth to approximately 6 months of age was the best single correlate ($r = 0.94271$) with the obesity score. The obesity score assigned to each child was based on a three-variable regression equation using weight gain, suprailiac skinfold, and waist circumference from the leanest and fattest children in the population, the leanest babies being assigned a score of 0 and the fattest babies a score of 1. Since weight gain was one of the variables used originally to establish the obesity score, it was not surprising to find that it correlated well. The only conclusion to be drawn from these data is that infants who are obese at 6 months of age most likely had a rapid weight gain since birth. Whether these infants remain obese at a later age is not known. It seems likely after careful scrutiny of Huenemann's population of infants that these are the identical subjects from Crawford' study. These infants were reevaluated at 3 years of age for weight status (weight:length:age) (60). Children were classified as overweight (greater than 110% of standard), normal (90 to 100% of standard), underweight (85 to 90% of standard), moderately protein-calorie malnourished (75 to 85% of standard), and severely protein-calorie malnourished (less than 75% of standard). Fourteen children were considered "fat" when 6 months of age. When restudied at age 3, five of the "fat" infants were overweight and nine were of normal weight. In general many of the 448 children in the study had shifted from one classification to another between 0.5 and 3 years of age.

Longer follow-up studies, using weight gain during the first 6 months of life to predict obesity, have also been reported. Eid reviewed birth records of all babies in a Sheffield, England hospital who had been born during a 1-year period (15). Infants who weighed more than 2500 g at birth, after a gestational period of 38 weeks or more, and had been followed up in the well-baby clinic at 6 weeks, 3 months, or 6 months, were selected for this study if their weight gain at one of the recorded follow-up points had been either rapid (weight gain above 90th percentile), average (weight gain around 50th percentile), or slow (weight gain below 10th percentile). From a total of 878 children born during this period, 224 were found to belong to one of the above weight gain groups and in addition were available for determination of body weight between the ages of 5 and 8 years. Children were considered overweight if their weight for height and sex was 10% above normal and obese if weight for height and sex was 20% above normal. A total of 20% of the children with a history of rapid weight gain in early infancy were greater than 10% above expected body weight compared to 9% of the children in the group with average weight gains and 6% in the slow weight gain groups. The author concluded that rapid weight gain in early infancy was a predictor of overweight and obesity persisting into later childhood. However, if this method was used exclusively, it is obvious that 80% of the rapid weight gain infants *would not* have become obese or overweight, and if they had been treated, presumably by food restriction, it would have been unnecessarily. Furthermore if rapid weight gain had been used as a criterion of overweight in the 224 subjects studied here, an incidence of 61% overweight (greater than 10% above expected weight) would have been expected, whereas the determined incidence was only 15%.

In another study 972 Swedish children, presumably representing the general Swedish population, were assessed for obesity (more than 20% above standard weight). Overweight between 10 and 20% above standard weight and weight gain during infancy were analyzed as possible predictors of later weight. Multiple regression analysis of the data indicated that only 10 to 20% of the variation in weight for height at 7 years could be explained by factors whose effect was detectable in infancy (54). Reports continue to be published for or against early weight gain or weight attained as a predictor of future weight status (61,62). Although predicting future body weight from weights recorded during infancy or from weight gains in infancy offers little practical application, it has been shown that the weight category a child has attained when 6 or 7 years old was similar to that attained when the child was restudied at age 13 or 14 (63). A similar correlation was seen when subjects studied at 10 to 13 years were reexamined as adults (64). Furthermore, although there is controversial evidence that some obesity in humans may be inherited, there is considerable consensus that obesity is a constellation of diseases, and that before we can assess the probability that some form of obesity is truly inherited we will have to develop a more meaningful classification of obesities. Fortunately, there are several strains of obese rodents in which the obesity is clearly inherited and in which development of the obesity can be sequentially studied. Furthermore, the relative modulations of nutritional and environmental factors on the development of the obesity can be assessed.

GENETIC OBESITY IN MICE

Among the obese rodents available for study are several mice strains shown in Table 4. The most widely studied of the obese mice are listed here. The obese hyperglycemic mouse ob/ob, inherits the obesity as a recessive gene (65). The obesity is of early onset, is characterized morphologically by both hyperplasia and hypertrophy of the adipose depot (66), and has elevated plasma immunoreactive insulin levels (67) and elevated plasma glucose levels (68,69), as well as numerous other metabolic changes. The diabetic mouse (db/db) also inherits its obesity as a recessive gene and the obesity is of early onset (70,71). The diabetic mouse is characterized by fat cell hypertrophy (66).

The yellow obese mouse (Ay/a) inherits the obesity in a fashion characteristic of a dominant trait (72,73). The homozygous dominant condition is apparently lethal, so that all obese yellow mice are, in fact, heterozygotes (74). The Ay/a mouse develops obesity later in life, the obesity is less severe, and it is characterized primarily by fat cellular hypertrophy (66). The remainder of the profile is characterized by a minor degree of hyperinsulinemia, no increase in plasma glucose levels, and only mildly elevated plasma lipids (75). There are several other strains of genetically obese mice that are less well studied, such as the adipose mouse (ad/ad) and the NZO mouse (75).

The various obese mice have been extremely helpful as models to study the fully developed obese condition. For example, much of the exciting work on insulin receptors has utilized the ob/ob mouse as a

Table 4   Mouse Obesities[a]

	Type	Age of Onset	Hypercellular	Hypertrophic	↑IRI	↑PG	↑TG
ob/ob	R	Early	Yes	Yes	Yes	Yes	Yes
db/db	R	Early	Slightly	Yes	No	Yes	Yes
A y/a	D	Late	No	Yes	Yes	No	Slightly

[a] IRI = immunoreactive insulin; PG = plasma glucose; TG = plasmatriglyceride; R = recessive gene; D = dominant gene.

Table 5   The Zucker Obese Rat (fa/fa) Model[a,b]

	fa/fa	Juvenile-Onset Obese
Excessive adipocity	Yes	Yes
Early onset	Yes	Yes
Hypercellular	Yes	Yes
Hypertrophic	Yes	Yes
↑IRI	Yes	Yes
↑TG	Yes	Yes
Normal PG	Yes	Yes
Skeletal retardation	Yes	No
Hypothalamic-hypophysiologic aberrations	Likely	Not likely

[a] From Gruen (96).
[b] IRI = immunoreactive insulin; TG = plasma triglyceride; PG = plasma glucose.

model (76–78). However, it is extremely difficult to utilize these mice to study the early postnatal development of the obesity or to manipulate factors early in growth because of the small size of the animal. As a consequence of the small organism size there are technical problems in attempting to deal with excessively small amounts of adipose tissue.

THE GENETICALLY OBESE ZUCKER RAT (fa/fa)

The discovery of the mutant "fatty" in a strain of rats derived from a cross of Sherman rats and Merck Stock M rats provided a much needed rat model for obesity. The Zucker obese rat inherits its obesity as a recessive trait (79). This particular rat has become increasingly popular as a model for juvenile-onset obesity in humans. It is, perhaps, not an entirely adequate model, particularly since in this rat, as well as in the ob/ob and Ay/a mouse strains, there is evidence of a disturbed hypothalamic-pituitary function (80). Nonetheless, the Zucker obese rat provides us with a genetic model to study experimentally which does have many characteristics in common with human obesity (Table 5).

The obesity of the Zucker rat can be readily identified in progeny at approximately 4 weeks of age, but not before. Homozygous recessive fatty females (fa/fa) do not mate, and only some homozygous fatty (fa/fa) males will mate. The two possible mating crosses are illustrated

Table 6   Possible Zucker Rat Matings

Fa/fa ♀ (heterozygous lean)	x ↓	fa/fa ♂ (homozygous fatty) predicted outcome
50% fa/fa (fatty)	+	50% Fa/fa (lean)
	or	
Fa/fa ♀ (heterozygous lean)	x ↓	Fa/fa ♂ (heterozygous lean) predicted outcome
25% Fa/Fa (lean)	+	50% Fa/fa + 25% fa/fa (lean) (fatty)

in Table 6. Recently techniques (81) have been developed, using the appropriate combination of food restriction and hormonal supplementation, which allow regular use of the mating between fa/fa males and heterozygous fa/fa females to produce progeny consisting of approximately 50% fatty pups. Previously, it was necessary to rely on the second mating, that is, matings of known heterozygote males and females to produce litters with an expected yield of 25% fatty pups. When litters of either crossings are examined there are no significant differences in body weight between rats which later become obese and their lean litter mates until at least the fourth postnatal week (Fig. 6). After this early postnatal period, the development sequence of the

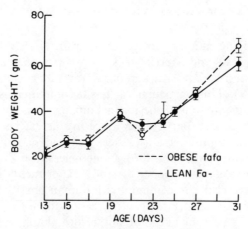

Figure 6.   Body weight accretion in lean and obese Zucker rats from 13 to 31 days of age (99).

obesity is more clearly apparent. By 5 weeks of age the obese rats are significantly heavier and become grossly obese as the animal continues to grow (82) (Fig. 7). It is clear that the increase in body weight is a case of increased adiposity from the standpoint of body composition. The obese rat has 20 to 30 times as much fat as its lean littermate when mature. This excessive adiposity is characterized by fat cell hypertrophy at all ages and by hyperplasia by 6 to 10 weeks of age, depending upon which site was examined (82).

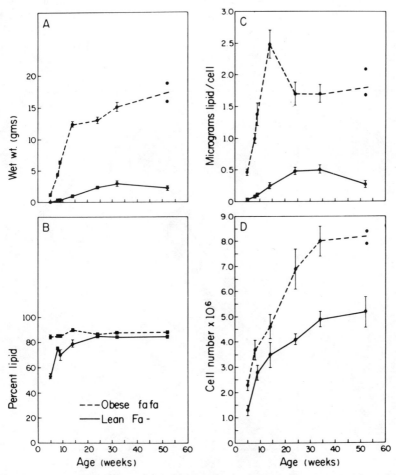

Figure 7. Adipose cellularity of the gonadal (i.e., parametrial) depot lean, female Zucker rats. (A) pad weights (B) percent lipid (C) adipose cell size and (D) adipose cell number (102).

The initial characterization of the developmental sequence of this obesity suggested that hypertrophy occurred first, and that hyperplasia occurred predominantly after the suckling period. It seemed, therefore, that early nutritional manipulation might prevent or at least modify this aspect of the obesity. Accordingly, rats were raised in litters of 4, 8, or 18 from birth until weaning, to produce three preweaning treatment groups: underfed, raised in litters of 15; standard fed, raised in litters of 8; and overfed, raised in litters of 4 (83). During the treatment period, the body weights of all rat pups were a reflection of the early dietary treatment. When all pups were weaned and allowed to eat ad libitum, the effectiveness of the early treatment was clearly modified (Fig. 8). While early nutritional experience plays a role in determining adult body weight, the obese trait is clearly expressed in all three fatty groups.

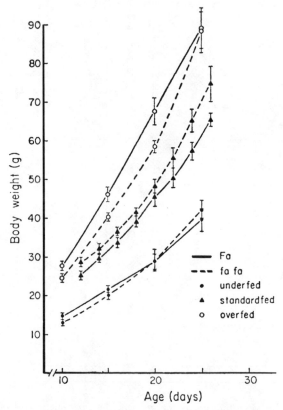

Figure 8. Preweaning growth of Zucker obese and nonobese rats. Effect of overnutrition and undernutrition (83).

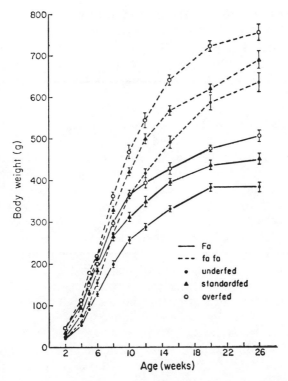

Figure 9. Postweaning groth of Zucker obese and nonobese rats. Effect of undernutrition and overnutrition during preweaning period (83).

All rats carrying the fatty trait weighed more than all lean rats. There is an effect of early nutritional experience in all three treatment groups but, clearly, the obese trait continues to be expressed (Fig. 9).

The normal lean littermate rat responds to early nutritional treatment as has been reported for other rat strains (84). Early undernutrition reduces fat cell number by about 20% while early overnutrition increased fat cell number by 20%. However, the fatty rats responded very differently. First, all fatty rats had more cells, and all had larger cells, than lean rats. Overfeeding during the suckling period increased fat cell number but underfeeding did not reduce fat cell number. Furthermore, chronic food restriction from birth to 15 weeks of age was also ineffective in preventing fat cell hyperplasia (85). These data suggest that fat cell proliferation remains unchecked in fatty rats and may be a primary defect in this genetic obesity. In our attempts to understand these inherited abnormalities of adipose tissue in rodents, we have attempted to conceptualize the development of normal adipose tissue. One of the major problems in studying the etiology of fat cell hyperplasia has been the inability to identify the precursor to the adipocyte. In any attempt to identify precursor cells, the definitive method available to modern cell biologists is to study the synthesis of DNA in these presumptive cells and to illustrate this by radioactively labeling the DNA of such cells during their replicative period. The use of this method to label DNA of precursor fat cells radioactively was pioneered by Hollenberg and Vost (86) and adapted by Greenwood and Hirsch (87) for further study. The data provided by these experiments have proved most useful in formulating a concept of how adipose tissue normally develops and suggested that in normal lean rats the hyperplastic period of growth in the epididymal fat pad occurs primarily during the first 4 to 6 weeks.

Although during normal growth adipose tissue mass attains a constant and stable proportion of the body's composition, it is clearly the case, in both human and rodent obesities, that considerable increments in adipose mass can be tolerated by the organism. This implies a certain flexibility in the system that makes adipose tissue unlike many other mammalian tissues, where doubling or tripling the amount of tissue would be lethal. Figure 10 presents a scheme for describing the regulation of adipose tissue mass during development. The concept suggested is common to a consideration of the developmental biology of

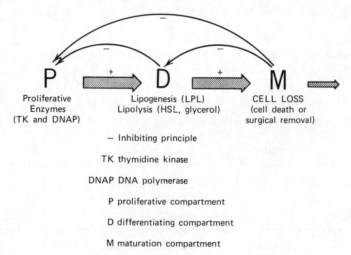

Figure 10.   A general scheme for adipose tissue mass regulation during development (103).

most organs. During early development, proliferation (P) predominates and cells once formed through mitotic activity move to the differentiation compartment (D), where they are induced to begin the accumulation of differentiation products. In the case of adipose tissue, of course, this is predominantly triglyceride (TG). As the cells accumulate sufficient TG, they move from D to the mature cell compartment (M), where they remain unless they die or are surgically removed. At least three regulatory feedback loops have been postulated in other systems and may be present in adipose tissue as well. A major signal is generated by the rate of enlargement of the M compartment, directly modulating compartment P. The M compartment also feeds back to regulate the rate of differentiation, or lipid filling of the cells, in the D compartment and D, in turn, feeds back to regulate P as well. In such a system the attainment of a present mature compartment size would generate a sufficient signal to suppress proliferation and stabilize the D compartment also. Such mechanisms and signals have been at least partially characterized in liver and skin.

What is the evidence that such a system could work in normal adipose tissue development? One way to stimulate proliferation would be to remove the mature compartment. Faust, Johnson, and Hirsch (88) have recently demonstrated that when this is done by surgical extirpation, or lipectomy, regeneration occurs. It occurs most easily when the tissue is removed at weaning, when the proliferative compartment is still most active. Surgical extirpation in 15-week-old rats results in no regeneration after 5 months as Kral has recently shown (89). Hence the data argue strongly for critical periods in the normal rat when cell proliferation can still be stimulated. The recent exciting developments in adipose cell culture add further evidence to this conceptualization work from the laboratories of Björntorp (90), and Roncari and Van (91) have indicated that precursor adipocytes can be encouraged to proliferate and differentiate in culture. Interestingly, in all cases in order to get demonstrable precursor cell growth, the mature cells, and presumably the inhibitory influences as well, must first be removed from the culture system.

ENZYMATIC STUDIES IN RAT ADIPOSE TISSUE

In order to study the relationship and regulation of these processes involved in proliferation, differentiation, and maturation, and to identify alteration that occurs in the development of genetic obesity, several enzymes associated with these compartments and stages of growth have been measured. The enzymes DNA polymerase (DNAP) and thymidine kinase (TK) were selected to monitor proliferation, since both have been shown to be well correlated with thymidine incorporation during hyperplastic growth of other tissues. In normal adipose tissue growth both of these enzymes show excellent agreement with the 3H thymidine incorporation data. Thymidine kinase is particularly well correlated, showing a high activity early and reaching adult levels of enzyme activity at 28 to 35 days (92), precisely the time when 3H thymidine incorporation also declined in normal tissue (Fig. 11). Thymidine kinase was measured in the developing genetically obese rat by Cleary et al. It was elevated from the earliest point measured, and remained elevated until 39 weeks of age (93). Although a primary abormality in the enzymes associated with proliferation might be postulated as a defect, this has seemed unlikely, since we have not been able to demonstrate appreciable hyperplasia in other tissues. Consequently, we felt that a study of the enzymes associated with cell enlargement and thus with the regulation of movement from the differentiation compartment might be useful.

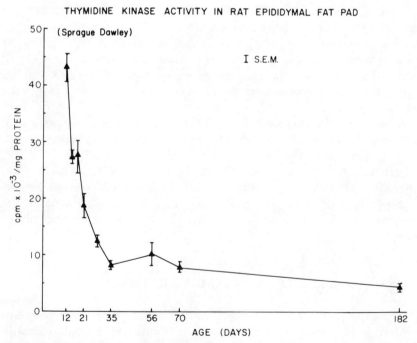

Figure 11. Thymidine kinase activity in normally growing Sprague-Dawley rat epididymal fat pads.

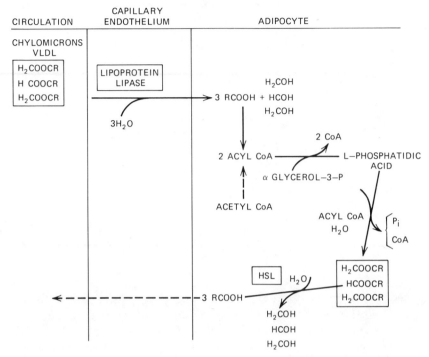

Figure 12. The role of lipoprotein lipase (LPL) in regulating fat cell triglyceride content.

Figure 12 indicates the manner in which lipoprotein lipase regulates the entrance of plasma FFA into the enlarging fat cell and how hormone-sensitive lipase and glycerol release reflect the breakdown of intracellular TG. The size of the fat cell might then be regarded as the net effect on these two systems. During normal development, LPL can be shown to increase before appreciable fat cell enlargement occurs (Fig. 13) (94). During early postnatal development LPL quadruples from 17 to 35 days, whereas fat cell size shows only small and not significant change. In the development of genetic obesity, an abnormality in the rate of lipid filling seemed even more likely to us, since it can be seen that cell size is increased in Zucker preobese rats as early as 5 days of age (95), and we can demonstrate elevated LPL/cell as early as 12 days of age when preobese Zucker rats are no heavier than their lean littermates (96). It seems feasible, then, that these very early changes in LPL activity do reflect a basic or at least a very early enzymatic disorder. It may be possible to rule out the hypothesis that suckling

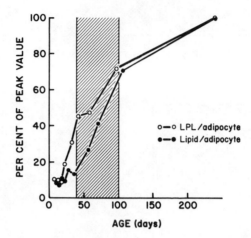

Figure 13. Lipoprotein lipase enzyme activity and fat cell size during the normal development of the rat epididymal fat pad (94).

genetically obese rats have a primary hyperphagic lesion and are ingesting more calories than needed. They do not weigh more than and are as active as lean sibs at least until 18 days of age (97). During the first 15 days of suckling, one can also be sure that the diet of lean and preobese pups is the same. Recent data using 3H labeled rat milk have demonstrated convincingly that the intake of obese and lean pups is comparable (98). Therefore, a dietary stimulus as the initiator of increased LPL activity seems unlikely. Many investigators have suggested that the primary initiating event in the development of obesity is a lesion in the β-cell, resulting in hypersecretion of insulin and elevated plasma IRI. Although early elevated IRI has been looked for in the Zucker rat, it has not been possible to demonstrate that elevated IRI precedes the obesity. Bell and Stern recently reported that they were unable to find differences in plasma IRI among rat pups at 13 days of age from breedings where 25% of the pups should have been preobese (99). Consequently, it remains a distinct and attractive possibility that changes in the regulation and synthesis of LPL may be a primary defect in the development of this form of genetic obesity in rodents.

THE OSBORNE-MENDEL RAT

In our consideration of animal models of obesity for use in developing testable hypotheses about the etiology of human obesity, we should also consider briefly the Osborne-Mendel rat. This rat, unlike the genetically obese Zucker rat, can remain thin for its entire life, unless the appropriate stimulus occurs. When this rat is allowed to eat a high fat or calorically dense diet it quickly becomes obese (100). The obesity is initially characterized by increased fat cell size, but after a "peak" fat cell size has been reached considerable fat cell hyperplasia occurs even in adult rats (101). The nature of the genetic defect in this rat is much less well understood and might be better described as a predisposition. Nonetheless, this type of obesity and this rat may provide a most useful model for studying late-onset hyperplastic obesity.

In conclusion, obesity is inherited in rodents both as a trait and as a genetic "predisposition." In the Zucker obese rat, an inborn error of metabolism may express itself early in development and lead to obesity even when hyperphagia is prevented. In most other rat strains the expression of the obesity is dependent upon environmental or nutritional stimulus. When a more useful classification of human obesities is formulated the use of these animal models to test hypotheses about the particular etiology of the obesities occurring in humans will be even more helpful.

REFERENCES

1. F. W. Lowenstein, *Bibl. Nutr.,* **26,** 154 (1978).
2. M. E. Moore, A. Stunkard, and L. Srole, *J.A.M.A.,* **181,** 962 (1962).
3. S. M. Garn, D. C. Clark, and K. E. Guire, "Growth, Body Composition, and Development of Obese and Lean Children," in M. Winick, Ed., *Childhood Obesity,* Wiley, New York, 1974, pp. 23–46.
4. A. Stunkard, E. D'Aquili, S. Fox, and R. D. L. Filion, *J.A.M.A.,* **221,** 579 (1972).
5. United States Government Printing Office, *Obesity and Fad Diets,* Apr. 12 (1973).
6. A. Shukla, H. A. Forsyth, C. M. Anderson, and S. M. Marwah, *Brit. Med. J.,* **Dec. 2,** 507 (1972).
7. J. L. Knittle and F. Ginsberg-Fellner, *Ped. Annals J.,* **258,** (1975).
8. M. L. Johnson, B. S. Burke, and J. Mayer, *Am. J. Clin. Nutr.,* **4,** 231 (1956).
9. M. C. Moore, A. Stunkard, and L. Srole, *J.A.M.A.,* **181,** 962 (1962).
10. J. Yudkin, J. Edelman, and L. Hough, London (1971).
11. L. S. Taitz, *Brit. Med. J.,* **Feb. 6,** 315 (1971).
12. L. S. Taitz, *Proc. Nutr. Soc.,* **33,** 113 (1974).
13. J. Mayer, P. Roy, and K. P. Mitra, *Am. J. Clin. Nutr.,* **4,** 169 (1956).
14. J. Mayer, *Postgrad. Med.,* **52,** 66 (1972).
15. E. E. Eid, *Brit. Med. J.,* **Apr. 11,** 74 (1970).

16. C. G. Neumann and M. Alpaugh, *Ped.*, **57**, 469 (1976).
17. S. M. Garn and D. C. Clark, *Ped.*, **57**, 443 (1976).
18. J. Mayer, Annals N. Y. Academy of Med., **131**, 142 (1965).
19. H. O. Mossberg, *Acta Paediatr.*, **35**, 21 (1948).
20. S. M. Garn, S. H. Bailey, and P. E. Cole, *Am. J. Physic. Anthrop.*, **45**, 539 (1976).
21. I. R. Shenker, V. Fisichelli, and J. Lang, *J. Ped.*, **84**, 715 (1974).
22. J. H. Newman, F. N. Freeman, and K. J. Holzinger, Univ. of Chicago Press (1937).
23. O. Von Verschuer, *Ergeb. inn. Med. Kinderheilk* **31**, 35 (1927).
24. H. Bakin, *Devel. Med. Child. Neurol.*, **15**, 178 (1973).
25. M. Borjeson, *Acta. Paediatr. Scand.*, **65**, 279 (1976).
26. C. G. D. Brook, R. M. C. Huntley, and J. Slack, *Brit. Med. J.*, **June 28**, 719 (1975).
27. J. Mayer, *Annals N.Y. Acad. of Sci.*, **63**, 15 (1955).
28. G. C. Kennedy, *Proc. Royal Soc.*, **140**, 578 (1953).
29. A. G. Mullins, *Arch. Dis. Child.*, **33**, 307 (1958).
30. J. Hirsch and J. L. Knittle, *Fed. Proc.*, **29**, 1516 (1970).
31. M. Krotkiewski, L. Sjostrom, P. Björntorp, G. Carlgren, G. Garellick, and U. Smith, *Int. J. Obesity*, **1**, 395 (1977).
32. J. Hirsch and B. Batchelor, *Clin. Endocrinol. Metab.*, **5**, 299 (1976).
33. P. Björntorp and L. Sjostrom, *Metab.*, **20**, 703 (1971).
34. G. Christakis, *Canad. J. Pub. Health*, **58**, 499 (1967).
35. A. Stunkard, H. Levine, and S. Fox, *Arch. Int. Med.*, **125**, 1067 (1970).
36. J. A. Glennon, *Arch. Int. Med.*, **118**, 1 (1966).
37. E. A. Sims, R. F. Goldman, M. Gluck, S. Horton, P. C. Kelleher, and D. W. Rowe, *Trans. Assoc. Am. Phys.*, **81**, 153 (1968).
38. C. G. D. Brook, *Lancet*, **Sept. 23**, 624 (1972).
39. C. G. D. Brook, J. K. Lloyd, and O. H. Wolf, *Brit. Med. J.*, **Apr. 1**, 25 (1972).
40. J. L. Knittle, *Triangle*, **13**, 57 (1974).
41. J. L. Knittle, *J. Ped.*, **81**, 1048 (1972).
42. J. Parizkova, *Proc. Nutr. Soc.*, **32**, 181 (1973).
43. J. Hirsch, *Postgrad. Med.*, **52**, 83 (1972).
44. D. Gairdner, *Proc. Nutr. Soc.*, **33**, 119 (1974).
45. J. L. Knittle, *N.Y. Acad. Med. Med. Bull.*, **47**, 579 (1971).
46. J. L. Knittle, F. Finsberg-Fellner, and R. E. Brown, *Am. J. Clin. Nutr.*, **30**, 762 (1977).
47. B. Forbes, *Ped.*, **34**, 308 (1964).
48. D. B. Cheek, B. Schultz, A. Parra, and R. C. Reba, *Ped. Res.*, **4**, 268 (1970).
49. J. K. Lloyd, O. H. Wolf, and W. S. Whelen, *Brit. Med. J.*, **July 15**, 145 (1961).
50. O. H. Wolf, *Quart. J. Med.*, **24**, 109 (1955).
51. J. Spranger and J. Dorken, *Nettsucht bei Kindern. Med. Mschr.*, **21**, 105 (1967).

52. R. A. Alley, J. V. Narduzzi, T. J. Robbins, T. F. Weir, G. Sabeh, and T. S. Danowski, *Clin. Ped.,* **7,** 112 (1968).

53. F. P. Heald and R. J. Hollander, *J. Ped.,* **67,** 35 (1965).

54. T. Melbin and J. C. Vuille, *Brit. J. Prev. Med.,* **27,** 225 (1973).

55. A. M. Bryans, *Canad. J. Pub. Health,* **58,** 486 (1967).

56. R. L. Huenemann, *J. Am. Diet. Assoc.,* **64,** 480 (1974).

57. G. S. Russel, R. Taylor, and C. E. Law, *Brit. J. Prev. Soc. Med.,* **22,** 119 (1968).

58. S. J. Fomon, L. N. Thomas, L. J. Filei, Jr., E. E. Ziegler, M. T. Leonard, *Acta. Paediatr. Scand.,* **223,** 1 (1971).

59. P. Crawford, C. A. Keller, M. C. Hampton, F. P. Pacheco, and R. L. Huenemann, *Am. J. Clin. Nutr.,* **27,** 706 (1974).

60. R. L. Huenemann, *J. Am. Diet. Assoc.,* **64,** 488 (1974).

61. G. Dorner, N. Hagen, and W. Witthuhn, *Acta. Biol. Med. Germ.,* **35,** 799 (1976).

62. E. Charney, H. C. Goodman, M. McBride, B. Lyon, and R. Pratt, *New Engl. J. Med.,* **295,** 6 (1976).

63. E. Sohar, E. Scapa, and M. Ravid, *Arch. Dis. Child.,* **48,** 389 (1973).

64. S. Abraham and M. Nordsieck, U.S. Pub. Health. Svc., Pub. Health Reports **75,** 263 (1960).

65. A. M. Ingalls, M. M. Dickie, and G. D. Snell, *J. Heredity,* **41,** 317 (1950).

66. P. R. Johnson and J. Hirsch, *J. Lipid Res.,* **13,** 2 (1972).

67. S. Westman, *Diabetologia,* **4,** 141 (1968).

68. H. F. P. Jooston and P. H. W. van der Kroon, *Metabolism,* **23,** 59 (1974).

69. V. R. Bileisch, J. Mayer, and M. M. Dickie, *Am. J. Path.,* **28,** 369 (1952).

70. K. Hummel, M. M. Dickie, and P. L. Coleman, *Science,* **153,** 1127 (1966).

71. D. L. Coleman and K. P. Hummel, *Diabetologia,* **3,** 238 (1967).

72. C. H. Danforth, *Proc. Soc. Exptl. Biol. Med.,* **24,** 69 (1926).

73. C. H. Danforth, *J. Heredity,* **18,** 153 (1927).

74. G. J. Eaton and M. M. Green, *Genetica,* **34,** 155 (1963).

75. G. A. Bray and D. A. York, *Physiol. Rev.,* **51,** 598 (1971).

76. Y. Marchand-Brustel, B. Jeanrenaud, and P. Freychet, *Am. J. Physiol.,* **234,** 348 (1978).

77. P. Freychet, M. H. Laudat, P. Laudat, G. Rosselin, C. R. Kahn, P. Gordon, and J. Roth, *FEBS Letter* **25,** 339 (1972).

78. M. P. Czech, D. K. Richardson, and C. J. Smith, *Progress in Endocrinology and Metabolism,* **1057** (1977).

79. L. M. Zucker and T. F. Zucker, *J. Heredity,* **52,** 275 (1961).

80. G. A. Bray, *Fed. Proc.,* **36,** 148 (1977).

81. R. B. Hemmes, S. Hubsch, and H. M. Pack, *Proc. Soc. Exp. Biol. Med.,* **159,** 424 (1978).

82. P. R. Johnson, L. M. Zucker, J. A. F. Cruce, and J. Hirsch, *J. Lipid Res.,* **12,** 706 (1971).

83. P. R. Johnson, J. S. Stern, M. R. C. Greenwood, L. M. Zucker, and J. Hirsch, *J. Nutr., 103*, 738 (1973).

84. J. L. Knittle and J. Hirsch, *J. Clin. Invest., 47*, 2091 (1968).

85. M. P. Cleary, J. R. Vasselli, C. Jen, and M. R. C. Greenwood, *Fed. Proc., 37*, 675 (1978).

86. C. H. Hollenberg and A. Vost, *J. Clin. Invest., 47*, 2485 (1968).

87. M. R. C. Greenwood and J. Hirsch, *J. Lipid Res., 15*, 474 (1974).

88. I. M. Faust, P. R. Johnson, and J. Hirsch, *Science, 197*, 391 (1977).

89. J. G. Kral, *Am. J. Physiol., 231*, 1090 (1976).

90. P. Björntorp, M. Karlsson, H. Pertoft, P. Pettersson, L. Sjostrom, and U. Smith, *J. Lipid Res., 19*, 316 (1978).

91. R. L. R. Van, C. E. Bayliss, and D. A. K. Roncari, *Clin. Invest., 58*, 699 (1976).

92. M. P. Cleary, B. E. Klein, M. R. C. Greenwood, and J. A. Brasel, *J. Nutr., 109*, In press.

93. M. P. Cleary, J. A. Brasel, and M. R. C. Greenwood, *Am. J. Physiol., 236*, in press.

94. E. Hietanen and M. R. C. Greenwood, *J. Lipid Res., 18*, 480 (1977).

95. A. Boulange, E. Planche, P. de Gasquet, and X. Leliepvre, Second International Congress on Obesity, Oct. (1977).

96. R. Gruen, E. Hietanen, and M. R. C. Greenwood, *Metabolism, 27* (12; Suppl 2), 1955 (1978).

97. J. S. Stern and P. R. Johnson, *Metabolism, 26*, 371 (1977).

98. A. Boulange, E. Planche, and P. de Gasquet, Second International Nutrition Congress, Oct., (1977).

99. G. E. Bell and J. S. Stern, *Growth, 41*, 63 (1977).

100. R. O. Schemmel, O. Mickelson, and J. L. Gill, *J. Nutr., 100*, 1041 (1970).

101. I. M. Faust, P. R. Johnson, J. S. Stern, and J. Hirsch, *Am. J. Physiol., 235*, E279 (1978).

102. P. R. Johnson, J. S. Stern, M. R. C. Greenwood, and J. Hirsch, *Metabolism, 27*(12, Suppl. 2) (1978).

103. M. R. C. Greenwood, R. Gruen, and M. P. Cleary, *Rec. Adv. Obesity Res., II* (1978).

PART 6

Hyperlipidemias

11

Human Mutations Affecting the Low Density Lipoprotein Pathway

MICHAEL S. BROWN and JOSEPH L. GOLDSTEIN

The Division of Medical Genetics, Department of Internal Medicine, University of Texas Health Science Center at Dallas, Dallas, Texas

An extensive series of biochemical and genetic studies over the past four years has defined the pathway by which extrahepatic human cells acquire the cholesterol that they need for plasma membrane synthesis (1). These studies, carried out primarily in cultured human fibroblasts, have revealed that when these cells are deprived of cholesterol they synthesize a specific plasma membrane receptor that binds the major cholesterol-carrying lipoprotein of human plasma, low density lipoprotein (LDL). Binding of LDL to the receptor is the first step in a pathway—the LDL pathway—by which cells take up the lipoprotein by endocytosis and utilize its cholesterol. By regulating the number of cell surface LDL receptors, cells are able to control the rate of entry of cholesterol, thereby assuring themselves an adequate supply of the sterol while at the same time preventing its overaccumulation. Since LDL is derived ultimately from the liver or intestine, the LDL pathway constitutes a mechanism by which cholesterol is transported to extrahepatic tissues from the liver (its site of synthesis) or the intestine (its site of absorption from the diet).

The American Journal of Clinical Nutrition 30: June 1977, pp. 975–978, Printed in U.S.A. Reproduced with permission. This work was supported by Grants from the National Foundation March of Dimes, the American Heart Association, and the National Institutes of Health (GM 19258 and HL 16024).

Michael S. Brown is Established Investigator of the American Heart Association. Joseph L. Goldstein is recipient of a Research Career Development Award from the National Institute of General Medical Sciences.

In order to utilize the cholesterol in plasma LDL, body cells bind the lipoprotein at the receptor site, internalize it by endocytosis and deliver it to lysosomes wherein the protein and cholesteryl ester components of the lipoprotein are hydrolyzed. The resulting free cholesterol is then available to be used by the cell for membrane synthesis. When sufficient cholesterol has accumulated to satisfy this requirement, three regulatory events occur: (1) cholesterol synthesis is turned off through a suppression of the rate-controlling enzyme, 3-hydroxy-3-methylglutaryl coenzyme A reductase (HMG CoA reductase); (2) excess lipoprotein-derived free cholesterol is reesterified for storage as cholesteryl esters through an activation of an acyl-CoA: Cholesterol acyltransferase; and (3) synthesis of the LDL receptor itself is diminished, thereby preventing further entry of LDL-cholesterol into the cell. These events in the LDL pathway are illustrated diagrammatically in Figure 1.

At each step in the delineation of the LDL pathway in cultured fibroblasts, interpretation of the data has been clarified by the analysis of mutant human fibroblasts derived from patients with genetic defects involving specific steps in the pathway. To date, six such mutations

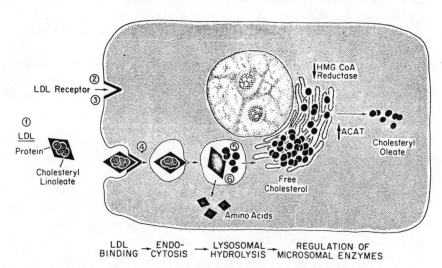

Fig. 1. Sequential steps in the LDL pathway in cultured human fibroblasts. The numbers indicate the sites at which mutations have been identified: (1) abetalipoproteinemia; (2) familial hypercholesterolemia, receptor-negative; (3) familial hypercholesterolemia, receptor-defective; (4) familial hypercholesterolemia, internalization defect; (5) Wolman syndrome; and (6) cholesteryl ester storage disease. HMG CoA reductase denotes 3-hydroxy-3-methylglutaryl coenzyme A reductase, and ACAT denotes acyl-coenzyme A: cholesterol acyltransferase. (Modified from (1)).

have been identified, five affecting the LDL pathway at the cellular level and one affecting the secretion of plasma LDL itself (2,3).

The mutation that has proved to have the greatest explanatory potential is the one found in patients with the homozygous form of receptor-negative familial hypercholesterolemia, an autosomal dominant disorder (mutation no. 2 in Fig. 1). The mutant fibroblasts from these homozygotes lack functional LDL receptors as determined by assays that are sufficiently sensitive to detect about 2% of the normal number. As a result, these cells fail to bind and take up the lipoprotein with high affinity and therefore fail to hydrolyze either its protein or cholesteryl ester components. Because they are unable to utilize LDL-cholesterol, these homozygote cells must satisfy their cholesterol requirement by synthesizing large amounts of cholesterol de novo, even when high levels of LDL are present in the culture medium. Moreover, in these mutant cells LDL does not stimulate the formation of cholesteryl esters.

In addition to the cells in which LDL receptor activity is not detectable (receptor-negative), a second class of mutant fibroblasts has been observed in which the maximal number of functional LDL receptors is reduced to about 5 to 20% of normal (mutation no. 3 in Fig. 1). Patients with this mutation have been designated as having the receptor-defective type of homozygous familial hypercholesterolemia. Both the receptor-defective and the receptor-negative mutations have been observed in fibroblasts obtained from subjects with the clinical phenotype of homozygous familial hypercholesterolemia. Such patients manifest extremely high levels of plasma LDL (their LDL-cholesterol levels are about 6 to 10 times normal), accumulation of free and esterified cholesterol in interstitial spaces and within phagocytic cells of the skin and tendons, and severe atherosclerosis with myocardial infarction occurring as early as 18 months of age.

The heterozygous parents of both the receptor-negative and receptor-defective homozygotes are more mildly affected than the homozygotes. These heterozygotes manifest plasma LDL levels that are 2 to 4 times the normal level and they usually develop clinical signs of atherosclerosis between the ages of 30 and 60. Fibroblasts from heterozygotes with the receptor-negative mutation have been shown to synthesize about one-half the normal number of LDL receptors and thus their cells take up and degrade LDL at one-half the normal rate. The consequences that the 50% deficiency in LDL receptors create for the regulation of cholesterol metabolism in this genetically dominant syndrome are reviewed elsewhere (4).

Recently, a third type of mutation in LDL uptake has been described in a patient who manifests a clinical syndrome indistinguishable from that of homozygotes with the receptor-negative and receptor-defective mutations (mutation no. 4 in Fig. 1). Fibroblasts from this patient are unique in that they are unable to internalize the receptor-bound lipoprotein. As a result, in these cells, just as in the cells from receptor-negative homozygotes, high affinity degradation of LDL does not occur and the lipoprotein does not suppress cholesterol synthesis nor does it stimulate cholesteryl ester formation. Since these mutant cells with the internalization defect resemble normal fibroblasts that have been treated with N-ethyl-maleimide, it has been postulated that they have a genetic defect not in the LDL binding site itself but in a sulfhydryl-containing protein that is necessary to mediate the internalization of receptor-bound LDL (3).

It is of interest that of 22 consecutively studied strains of fibroblasts derived from patients in 11 countries who manifest the clinical phenotype of classic homozygous familial hypercholesterolemia, 12 were found to be receptor-negative, nine were receptor-defective, and one exhibited the internalization defect (Table 1).

In addition to the three known mutations that produce the syndrome of familial hypercholesterolemia, two other mutations have been shown to affect the LDL pathway in fibroblasts. These mutations (mutations no. 5 and no. 6 in Fig. 1) occur in patients with the Wolman syndrome and cholesteryl ester storage disease, two autosomal recessive disorders in which cholesteryl esters accumulate abnormally in lysosomes of cells throughout the body. Studies by Patrick and Lake (5) disclosed that the primary defect in the Wolman syndrome involves the absence of a lysosomal acid lipase that normally hydrolyzes both cholesteryl esters and triglycerides. In the related, but clinically less severe syndrome of cholesteryl ester storage disease, the activity of this same lysosomal acid lipase is reduced to about 1 to 5% of normal (6). When incubated with

Table 1   Biochemical Analysis of Fibroblast Strains Derived from 22 Subjects with the Clinical Syndrome of Homozygous Familial Hypercholesterolemia

Biochemical Phenotype	No. of Subjects
Receptor-negative	12
Receptor-defective	9
Internalization defect	1

LDL, fibroblasts from patients with both of these disorders bind and take up the lipoprotein normally and degrade its protein component at a normal rate. However, the defect in lysosomal acid lipase activity prevents normal hydrolysis of the cholesteryl ester component of LDL. As a result the cholesteryl esters of LDL accumulate within lysosomes and the lipoprotein fails acutely to suppress HMG CoA reductase or to activate the acyl-CoA: cholesterol acyltransferase (1).

Clinically, in the Wolman syndrome the absence of the lysosomal acid lipase produces a massive accumulation of cholesteryl esters and triglycerides in nearly all body tissues and death ensues within the first year of life. In cholesteryl ester storage disease, the residual acid lipase activity is sufficient to allow survival to young adulthood. It is of importance that in the few of these young patients whose tissues have been studied at autopsy cholesteryl ester accumulation was particularly marked in the arterial wall and advanced atherosclerosis was noted (6).

Another mutation that has proved useful in working out the LDL pathway is the one that produces the autosomal recessive disease abeta-lipoproteinemia (mutation no. 1 in Fig. 1). This genetic defect causes a block in either the synthesis or the secretion of apo-protein B, so that the plasma of these patients is devoid of LDL. Although their plasma contains cholesterol bound to other lipoproteins (mainly HDL), this cholesterol cannot be taken up by normal fibroblasts in tissue culture and hence it fails to suppress HMG CoA reductase activity or to stimulate cholesteryl ester formation in normal cells. These observations have been used to support the conclusion that only those human cholesterol-carrying lipoproteins that contain apoprotein B—namely, LDL and VLDL—are able to bind the LDL receptor and deliver cholesterol to fibroblasts.

All of the steps of the LDL pathway in human fibroblasts have also been observed to occur in long term human lymphoid cells in suspension culture and in human aortic smooth muscle cells in monolayer culture. In particular, studies by Kayden et al. (7) and Ho et al. (8) have established that cholesterol synthesis and esterification in lymphoid cells are regulated through the LDL receptor. More important, these investigators have also shown that lymphoid cells from patients with the receptor-negative form of homozygous familial hypercholesterolemia lack cell surface LDL receptors and therefore exhibit the same constellation of secondary defects (i.e., defective LDL uptake and degradation, overproduction of cholesterol, and failure to induce cholesteryl ester formation) as do the receptor-negative homozygote fibroblasts.

Of particular relevance to atherosclerosis are the studies on the regulation of the LDL pathway in cultured human aortic smooth muscle cells. These studies have demonstrated that aortic smooth muscle cells, like fibroblasts, regulate the number of LDL receptors so as to take up and degrade only enough LDL to supply cellular needs for cholesterol. Because of this regulation, the addition of large amounts of native LDL to smooth muscle cells in culture does not induce an overaccumulation of cholesteryl esters of the type that is observed in the atherosclerotic lesion in vivo (9).

It is clear that further studies of the properties of the LDL pathway in various tissues should provide additional insight into the normal mechanisms by which specific cells regulate their cholesterol metabolism. These studies should also reveal the manner in which these genetic control mechanisms are perturbed by the nutritional stresses as well as other stresses that produce atherosclerosis in western man.

REFERENCES

1. M. S. Brown, and J. L. Goldstein. *Science,* **191,** 150 (1976).
2. M. S. Brown, and J. L. Goldstein, *New Engl. J. Med.,* **294,** 1386 (1976).
3. M. S. Brown, and J. L. Goldstein. *Cell,* **9,** 663 (1976).
4. D. S. Fredrickson, J. L. Goldstein, and M. S. Brown, "The familial hyperlipoproteinemias," In J. B. Stanbury, J. B. Wyngaarden, and D. S. Fredrickson, Eds., *The Metabolic Basis of Inherited Disease,* 4th ed., McGraw-Hill, New York, in press.
5. A. D. Patrick, and B. D. Lake, "Wolman's disease," in H. G. Hers and F. Von Hoof, Eds., *Lysosomes and Storage Diseases,* Academic, New York, 1973, pp. 453–73.
6. H. R. Sloan, and D. S. Fredrickson, "Rare familial diseases with neutral lipid storage: Wolman's disease, cholesteryl ester storage disease, and cerebrotendinous xanthomatosis," in: J. B. Stanbury, J. B. Wyngaarden and D. S. Fredrickson, Eds., *The Metabolic Basis of Inherited Disease,* McGraw-Hill, New York, 1972, pp. 808–832.
7. H. J. Kayden, L. Hatam, and N. G. Beratis, *Biochemistry,* **15,** 521 (1976).
8. Y. K. Ho, M. S. Brown, H. J. Kayden and J. L. Goldstein. *J. Exptl. Med.,* **144,** 444 (1976).
9. J. L. Goldstein, and M. S. Brown. *Ann. Rev. Biochem.,* **46,** 897 (1977).

12

Nutrition Management
of Hyperlipidemias

WILLIAM E. CONNOR, M.D. and
SONJA L. CONNOR, M.S., R.D.

Divisions of Metabolism-Nutrition and Cardiology, The Department of Medicine,
University of Oregon Health Sciences Center, Portland, Oregon

There are four important clinical reasons for concern about hyperlipidemia. The first reason is the strong correlation between hypercholesterolemia and atherosclerotic disease of the heart, brain, viscera, and legs. The control and prevention of atherosclerosis in our population depends largely on lowering plasma cholesterol and low density lipoprotein (LDL) levels (1).

The second reason relates to the occurrence of xanthomas in the skin, tendons, eyelids, and in various internal ecotopic locations. Xanthomas are usually, but not always, related to elevated plasma lipid levels. Their significance is not only cosmetic; often they are of diagnostic significance, suggesting the presence of an underlying blood abnormality and, at times, its nature.

Third, hyperlipidemia must also be considered in patients with abdominal pain. As was pointed out years ago, such patients may have hyperchylomicronemia and hypertriglyceridemia. The episodes of abdominal pain are directly related to the hyperlipidemia, the correction of which will lead to the relief of these symptoms (2). In many instances the episodes of abdominal pain may proceed to acute hemorrhagic pancreatitis. The situation leads to the clinical dictum that all patients with acute pancreatitis should subsequently be screened for the presence

Supported by U.S. Public Health Service Grants from the National Heart, Lung, and Blood Institute (HL-20910) and from the General Clinical Research Centers Program (RR 334) of the Division of Research Resources of the National Institutes of Health.

of hyperlipidemia, since acute pancreatitis is especially common in patients with types I and V hyperlipidemia. This life-threatening problem may be prevented in the future only by the appropriate dietary treatment of the hyperlipidemic state.

Finally, as the fourth reason for concern, the presence of hyperlipidemia may point to the presence of another disease, such as hypothyroidism, poorly controlled diabetes mellitus, renal disease, biliary obstruction, and many others. All of these clinical points attest to the need for nutritional management of hyperlipidemia, the focal point for discussion in this chapter.

A summary of the specific pathology related to the various plasma lipids and lipoproteins follows. Hypercholesterolemia represented by low density lipoprotein (LDL) (type II) leads to atherosclerosis and xanthomas. Hypertriglyceridemia with excessive chylomicrons (types I and V) causes episodes of abdominal pain and acute pancreatitis, and, in addition, eruptive xanthomata of the skin. Hypertriglyceridemia with increased VLDL, or IDL or both (types IV, II-b and III) may be involved in both atherosclerosis and xanthomata. In a rare genetic disease, β-sitosterolemia and xanthomatosis, plant sterols are present in the blood and give rise to xanthoma formation where plasma cholesterol levels are normal.

Hyperlipidemic states represent some of the most common entities seen in the practice of medicine and are among the most common genetic abnormalities seen in our population. Furthermore, depending on where cutoff points are drawn, one-third to one-half of Americans of all ages have mild to severe hyperlipidemia. This makes the condition exceptionally common, even more ingrained in Americans than a recognized common entity such as essential hypertension. Thus, hyperlipidemia represents a vast arena for the application of very sophisticated preventive medicine, with emphasis on the primary role of nutrition. Most hyperlipidemic patients will have had the disorder for years before any discrete clinical manifestations appear. Furthermore, once hyperlipidemia develops, the condition is usually permanent unless appropriate treatment is provided.

The cornerstone in the treatment of hyperlipidemia is dietary alteration (3). This is true regardless of the degree to which primary genetic abnormalities are partly or completely responsible for the development of the hyperlipidemia. Dietary factors in the American population inevitably exacerbate any genetic abnormality that may be largely responsible for the hyperlipidemic state, and dietary treatment will almost always result in some improvement in the condition. Therapy has been simplified by the concept that a single basic diet may be used initially in the treatment of all forms of hyperlipidemia. The design of the single diet incorporates current research results with regard to the specific dietary constituents that affect plasma lipid and lipoprotein concentrations, as will be reviewed subsequently. The single diet is low in cholesterol and low in total and saturated fat; it is high in complex carbohydrate. It is of low caloric density and provides calories only sufficient to achieve and maintain ideal body weight.

The aim of the dietary treatment of hyperlipidemia is straightforward: it is the achievement of normal plasma cholesterol, triglyceride, and lipoprotein concentrations when possible in order to (1) prevent and treat atherosclerosis of the coronary arteries and of the other arteries of the body; (2) prevent episodes of abdominal pain and acute pancreatitis; and (3) correct and prevent xanthomatous deposits in the skin and tendons. Dietary treatment should be initiated when the plasma cholesterol concentration is above 200 mg/dl in older adults and 180 mg/dl in young adults and children. The upper limit for plasma triglyceride concentration is 140 mg/dl.

The recommended dietary treatment is appropriate and safe for both adults and children. Such dietary treatment must clearly answer all the nutritional needs of the body and at the same time have beneficial effects upon the elevated plasma lipid and lipoprotein concentrations. Both of these criteria have been answered both theoretically and practically (3,4).

THE EFFECTS OF SPECIFIC NUTRIENTS ON THE PLASMA LIPIDS AND LIPOPROTEINS

Historically, and to the present time, a vast amount of evidence in both man and animals has indicated that a certain dietary factors have hyperlipidemic effects (Table 1). Many other factors have minimal effects or none at all. Two groups of substances while consumed almost as pharmaceutical agents are hypolipidemic (pectin, polyunsaturated fat), but have certain potential side effects or difficulties of administration which would make their use in the "single diet" of limited value. All of these nutritional factors will be discussed in detail to provide both a theoretical and a practical basis for the all-important dietary prescription in the treatment of hyperlipidemia. It is hoped that this discussion will simplify the problem of dietary management for the physician responsible for the care of the hyperlipidemic patient.

Table 1   The Effects of Various Dietary Factors on the Plasma Lipids in Man

Hyperlipidemic dietary factors
   1. Dietary cholesterol
   2. Saturated fat
   3. Total fat
   4. Total calories
   5. Alcohol (in some individuals only)

Hypolipidemic dietary factors
   6. Polyunsaturated fat (in very high amounts)[a]
   7. Some fibers (pectin, guar gum)

Dietary factors with no discrete long term effects
   8. Carbohydrate
   9. Most fibers
   10. Protein
   11. Vitamins and minerals

[a] Very high amounts of polyunsaturated fat while resulting in a hypocholesterolemic effect overall would produce postprandial hypertriglyceridemia.

Cholesterol

Cholesterol has an important effect upon lipid metabolism (4). In 1912, it was identified as the constituent of animal foods which would readily elevate the serum cholesterol levels and produce atherosclerosis in experimental animals. Subsequently, cholesterol-rich diets have regularly caused hypercholesterolemia, atherosclerosis, and even, at times, myocardial infarction in a large number of species of experimental animals, including primates (5). The regression of atherosclerosis in primates has routinely occurred when the cholesterol-containing diet was replaced by a cholesterol-free diet which lowered the plasma cholesterol level greatly (6).

By the early 1960s, a decisive effect of dietary cholesterol on the serum lipid levels in humans was clearly demonstrated in a series of metabolic ward experiments carried out in normal volunteers (7–11). Figures 1 and 2 depict the results of two such studies, one lasting for almost a year and the other for a 12-week period (4,8). Dietary cholesterol invariably elevated the plasma cholesterol and phospholipid concentrations when fed as egg yolk in balanced diets preceded by a cholesterol-free dietary period. The plasma cholesterol levels declined with the subsequent removal of dietary cholesterol. The amounts of die-

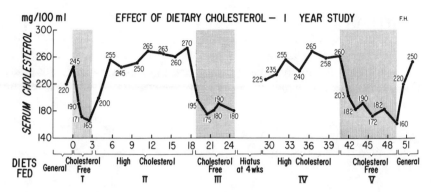

Figure 1. The effects of dietary cholesterol upon the serum cholesterol levels in a 34-year-old man over a 12-month period. The diets of mixed, general foods were either cholesterol free or contained 2400 mg of cholesterol supplied by egg yolk. In both diets, the protein was 15% of total calories, the fat 40% (14% saturated, 17% monounsaturated, and 10% polyunsaturated), and carbohydrate 45%. The iodine number of the dietary fat in all diets was 80 to 85. The calories were adjusted to maintain a constant body weight.

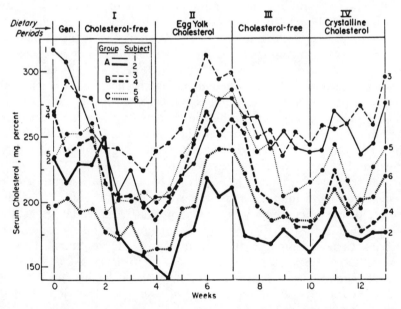

Figure 2. The serum cholesterol values for each subject during the different dietary periods. In period II, group A subjects received 475 mg, group B 950 mg, and group C 1425 mg of egg yolk cholesterol. In period IV, group A subjects received 1200 mg of crystalline cholesterol, group B 2400 mg, and group C 3600 mg.

183

tary cholesterol ranged from 475 mg/day upward. The increase in plasma cholesterol in these studies ranged from +69 mg/dl to +80 mg/dl. The changes in plasma cholesterol from the addition or removal of dietary cholesterol in the above diets were persistent. In the one study (Fig. 2), the mean plasma cholesterol levels were 191 ± 8.5 (SE) for the cholesterol-free diet and 260 ± 4.3 for the high cholesterol diet, highly significant differences. Amounts of dietary cholesterol from 475 to 1425 mg/day had similar effects, suggesting a ceiling effect of cholesterol intake beyond which no further increment in plasma cholesterol occurred.

Dietary cholesterol is absorbed by the gut in amounts proportional to the intake up to a dietary level of perhaps 1200 to 1500 mg/day. Only about 40% of the intake is absorbed (12). In man, absorbed cholesterol is transported initially in chylomicrons largely as ester cholesterol, reaches a peak concentration in the plasma some 48 hours after a given meal, and then contributes its mass to the total body pools of cholesterol (13). Cholesterol-rich chylomicron remnants are then metabolized by the liver.

Cholesterol of dietary origin is transferred ultimately into other lipoprotein classes, especially beta or low density lipoproteins (LDL), and contributes in this manner to elevations of the total plasma cholesterol as is shown in the following study (14). Twenty-five subjects who had been previously consuming the usual American diet were given cholesterol-free diets for 3 to 4 weeks and then 1000 mg/day of dietary cholesterol were incorporated into their diets for another 3 to 4 weeks. The diets were otherwise identical and contained 40% of the calories as fat. All subjects had a pronounced decline in plasma cholesterol concentrations following the consumption of the cholesterol-free diet (Table 2). The previous typical American diet had been high in cholesterol and saturated fat. The mild and severe type II-a, the type IV, and the normal subjects responded similarly. The composite mean level of plasma cholesterol for the 25 subjects was 211 mg/dl with the baseline cholesterol-free diet. Egg yolk cholesterol (1000 mg/day) was then incorporated into the diet without changing the other constituents (calories, carbohydrate, fat, protein, minerals, and vitamins). This egg yolk cholesterol increased the plasma cholesterol level to 247 mg/dl, or a net change of +36 mg/dl. All subjects changed in the upward direction, even the type IV subjects. The severe type II subjects had the greatest change, an increase of 67 mg/dl.

The crucial problem of this study was then to ascertain which lipoprotein fractions had changed in response to the 1000 mg high cholesterol diet. The high cholesterol diet increased not only the total plasma

Table 2 The Plasma Cholesterol Levels (mg/dl) after the Usual American Diet and Cholesterol-Free and High-Cholesterol Diets in Normal and Hyperlipoproteinemic Subjects

	Usual American Diet	Period I		Period II		
		Cholesterol-free Diet	Change	Cholesterol-free Diet	High Cholesterol Diet	Change
Normal subjects	171 ± 8 (SD)	141 ± 14	−30	141 ± 14	174 ± 20	+33
Type II-a mild	258 ± 18	209 ± 27	−49	209 ± 27	245 ± 29	+36
Type II-a severe	375 ± 22	338 ± 43	−38	338 ± 43	405 ± 17	+67
Type IV	251 ± 36	208 ± 23	−43	208 ± 23	231 ± 23	+23
Means of all subjects				211 ± 68	247 ± 79	+36

185

cholesterol concentration but also certain lipoprotein fractions. For normal subjects and those with type II-a hyperlipidemia, the increase occurred almost entirely in the form of LDL lipoprotein, with slight increases in alpha or high density lipoprotein (HDL) (Fig. 3). There are no significant increases in very low density lipoprotein (VLDL). In the type IV patients, however, a somewhat different result occurred. Both VLDL and LDL cholesterol increased. Each accounted for about 50% of the total increase. But, for most individuals, the effects of dietary cholesterol were reflected in an increased LDL cholesterol concentration. This pertains even to normal subjects with quite low baseline plasma cholesterol levels (141 mg/dl) as well as to the type II-a subjects with mild or severe hypercholesterolemia.

In addition, it is apparent from the data that HDL cholesterol also increased after the ingestion of dietary cholesterol. Mahley and colleagues have indicated in both animals and man that the HDL increase is in the form of HDL_c, which cannot be regarded as a beneficial form of HDL (15). The composition of HDL_c is quite different from the usual HDL present before feeding the dietary cholesterol. The chief compositional change is enrichment of HDL with arginine-rich apoproteins and a tremendous amount of cholesterol ester. These characteristics make HDL_c more analogous in many ways to LDL, which also has a large quantity of cholesterol ester, than to the usual

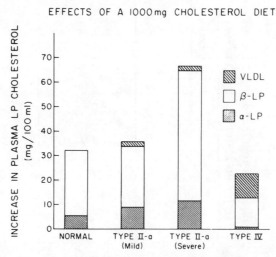

Figure 3. The effects of a 1000 mg cholesterol diet upon the plasma lipoproteins in 25 subjects. The baseline diet which preceeded the 1000 mg cholesterol diet was virtually a cholesterol-free diet.

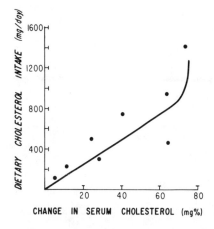

Figure 4.   The effects of different intakes of dietary cholesterol upon the serum cholesterol levels in men. The baseline diets in all instances were virtually cholesterol free.

HDL. This interesting work would suggest that such an HDL_c might even be atherogenic, as is LDL, because it also induces the uptake of cholesterol ester in tissue culture cells, which the normal HDL does not do.

Another question that arises is, what is the threshold amount of dietary cholesterol necessary to produce an increase in total plasma cholesterol concentration? For example, in the study already quoted (Fig. 2), 475 mg of cholesterol, or the equivalent of approximately two egg yolks per day, definitely caused an increment of some 60 mg/dl of plasma cholesterol in individuals previously consuming a cholesterol-free diet. But the use of 950 and 1425 mg/day produced no greater effects than the 475. Figure 4 illustrates this concept of threshold. For many people the threshold may be between 200 and 500 mg/day of dietary cholesterol. Thus, if subjects are eating over 500 mg/day, the addition of further dietary cholesterol would not change plasma cholesterol concentration (13). Our concept is also that the addition of 100 mg/day of dietary cholesterol to individuals previously consuming a cholesterol-free diet did not have any effect upon plasma cholesterol concentration, whereas 300 mg/day certainly did have (16).

The mechanism whereby dietary cholesterol increases the total plasma cholesterol concentration and also LDL cholesterol concentration may be related to an overload of the disposal system for sterols. This may be illustrated by the sterol balance concept (Table 3). The input of sterols into the plasma–tissue pool is twofold: from dietary cholesterol (0 to 1500 mg/day) and from cholesterol synthesized by the liver and gut. The synthesis rate of cholesterol in man is not very labile; most studies have shown little effect upon synthesis from ingestion of

Table 3   The Cholesterol Balance of the Body

Input	
From synthesis	500–1000 mg/day
Absorbed from the diet	0–400 mg/day
	500–1400 mg/day
Output	
Excretion in the bile (cholesterol and bile acids) and subsequently in the feces	400–1300 mg/day
Skin excretion	80–100 mg/day
Synthesis of steroid hormones	variable
Losses during pregnancy and lactation	variable
Storage in the tissues	variable
	500–1400 mg/day

dietary cholesterol. This means that the total amount of sterol entering the body either from diet or by synthesis will be much greater in individuals consuming a high cholesterol diet than in individuals consuming a low cholesterol diet. The output of sterols from the body is largely via the feces and includes the cholesterol and bile acids excreted in the bile and not reabsorbed by the gut. Most studies to date have indicated a failure of bile acid and neutral steroid excretion to increase very much after the ingestion of dietary cholesterol. Thus, two consequences may result from the ingestion of dietary cholesterol. The first is a rise in plasma cholesterol concentration. The second, a direct consequence of the first, is the ultimate deposition of increased amounts of cholesterol in the tissue, particularly in the arteries, to initiate and sustain the atherosclerotic process.

Dietary Fat, Amount and Saturation

The amounts and kinds of fat in the diet have well-documented effects on the plasma lipid concentrations (17,18). The amount of fat in a meal directly affects chylomicron formation in the gut mucosa and results in the postprandial elevation of plasma triglyceride. Thus, with defects in triglyceride clearances which occur in types I and V hyperlipidemia, it is essential to reduce the amount of dietary fat to a level that does not leave residual chylomicrons in the fasting plasma. The imperative rationale for the decrease in total dietary fat, then, is to avoid episodes of abdominal pain and pancreatitis and to reduce the formation of chylomicron remnants, these being atherogenic particles. After the ingestion of a meal rich in fat, the plasma triglyceride (carried by chylomicrons) increases from the fasting level, whatever it may be, to a peak in normal individuals at 3 to 5 hours, with a decrease to baseline by 7 hours. With the defects of clearance seen in types I and V, postprandial hypertriglyceridemia may persist for 12 to 24 hours or even days.

Regardless of baseline plasma lipid levels, the ingestion of 25 to 75 g of fat or sometimes even smaller amounts in a meal will lead to the chylomicron formation and the discharge of chylomicrons. Mild chylomicronemia is clearly physiologic. However, its intensity and duration have been considered possible factors in the pathogenesis of atherosclerosis since the 1940s. Recent evidence indicates that the chylomicron itself is probably not the culprit in the atherogenic propensity that postprandial lipemia may have. Instead, a product of chylomicron metabolism called the chylomicron remnant may possibly be the injurious agent (19). Remnants have been categorized in many species and are rich in both triglyceride and cholesterol and have a much smaller size than chylomicrons. Recognizable remnant particles include those found in abundance in rabbit plasma after the feeding of cholesterol and fat and those found in the type III (IDL) abnormality. Thus, we postulate that the more intense the postprandial lipemia, the greater will be remnant formation and thus the greater the effect upon the atherogenic process. Remnants may be viewed in many individuals as directly proportional to the amount of dietary fat ingested each day.

While large amounts of dietary fat may enhance dietary cholesterol absorption, and hence increase plasma cholesterol levels, the most important direct effect of dietary fat on plasma cholesterol levels is related to the type of fat. Saturated fat in the diet elevates and polyunsaturated fat depresses plasma cholesterol levels. Monounsaturated fat (oleic acid being the characteristic fatty acid) has a neutral effect and does not in itself either elevate or depress the plasma lipids. All animal fats are highly saturated except those derived from fish and shellfish, which are contrastingly highly unsaturated. Many, but not all, of the currently marketed vegetable oils, shortenings, and margarines are only lightly hydrogenated and thus retain the basic unsaturated characteristics of vegetable oils in general. Coconut oil, cocoa butter (the fat of chocolate), and palm oil are common saturated vegetable fats consumed in quantities; they have a hypercholesterolemic effect. The ratio of polyunsaturated to saturated fatty acids in a given fat or oil is termed the P/S value. Fats with a high P/S value of 2 and above are generally recognized as being hypocholesterolemic; those with P/S values of 0.4 or less are hypercholesterolemic. The typical American diet has a P/S value of 0.4 In therapeutic diets, the P/S value is 1.0 or above.

Most comparisons of the effects of saturated and polyunsaturated fat on plasma lipids have indicated that the plasma cholesterol elevating effect of saturated fat, gram for gram, is up to two times greater than the plasma cholesterol depressing effect of polyunsaturated fat (18,19). Regression equations have been calculated to indicate the plasma cholesterol changes from dietary manipulations of saturated fat, polyunsaturated fat, and cholesterol. One such equation (18) which fits our own experiences best is

$$\Delta \text{Chol} + 2.16 \text{ S} - 1.65 \text{ P} + 6.77 \text{ C} - 0.53$$

where Δ Chol = the change in plasma cholesterol (mg/dl)

ΔS = the change in saturated fat as per cent of total calories

ΔP = the change in polyunsaturated fat as per cent of total calories

C = dietary cholesterol intake (dg/day)

Pronounced cholesterol lowering effects from dietary polyunsaturated fat have invariably resulted only if the changes in dietary fat composition were drastic, usually in a metabolic ward situation where precisely calculated diets could be utilized. These circumstances seldom pertain to real life. For example, in one typical study, the dietary induced changes in serum lipids occurred when corn oil was the sole source of fat (40% of total calories) as compared to cocoa butter (22). The P/S fatty acid comparisons were 4.7 for the corn oil diet and 0.05 for the cocoa butter diet. The serum cholesterol declined 29% with the corn oil feeding. Such a great dietary difference would not be possible for free living patients to follow.

Because of the spectacular results from metabolic ward experiments, efforts have been made to increase the amount of polyunsaturated fat in the diet of free living hyperlipidemic patients. At times there has been an almost pharmacological use of vegetable oils to promote the lowering of plasma lipid levels. However, the single diet concept for the treatment of hyperlipidemia does not advocate an increase in polyunsaturated fat over what most Americans are already consuming. There have been a number of important reasons for this deliberate omission. There is no historical precedent for the diets of human beings to have a linoleic acid content (this being the chief fatty acid of most polyunsaturated vegetable oils) of more than 6 to 8% of the total calories; such a level is already the characteristic intake of many Americans at present. While the fatty acid composition of all body membranes is changed by a diet high in polyunsaturated fat in the direction of more linoleic acid content, there is simply no information that such changes over the lifetime would be harmless. However, some harmful effects of polyunsaturated fat have already been described. These include enhanced formation of gallstones (23), increased vitamin E requirements, the promotion of obesity, an increase in intake of plant sterols, and a possible increase of cholesterol adsorption. The issue of whether polyunsaturated fat in the diet might also be a stimulus to carcinogenesis is still unsettled (24).

With regard to weight control, the use of large quantities of polyunsaturated vegetable oils poses a serious problem because any fat is such a calorically dense foodstuff. A high fat diet is undoubtedly a major contributor to the excessive calories ingested by the obese. Adding tablespoons of polyunsaturated oils to the recipes of the presumed cholesterol lowering diet or simply taking oil straight would add a great many calories to the diets of patients whose chief problem may be weight control.

Since the amount of total fat in the diet, regardless of kind, may be of importance in promoting cholesterol adsorption and also definitely contributes to the flux of lipid through the blood in the form of chylomicrons and the subsequent remnant particles, there are sound theoretical reasons for keeping the total fat reduced in diets designed for the treatment of hyperlipidemia. The total dietary fat must, of course, be kept low for the treatment of types I and V hyperlipidemia. A low total fat intake will keep to a minimum the formation of atherogenic chylomicron remnants, as has already been stressed. Finally, if appropriate measures are taken to lower dietary cholesterol and saturated fat, then pronounced lowering of plasma cholesterol levels may be obtained without adding polyunsaturated fat to the diet. For all of these reasons, the prescription in the single diet for the treatment of hyperlipidemia is a reduction of dietary fat to 20% of the total calories, and most of this reduction is in the form of saturated fat. Polyunsaturated fat is simply not increased above 6 to 8% of the total calories.

Calories

The excessive caloric consumption of any food source which leads to adiposity may also result in hypertriglyceridemia in many susceptible individuals. This may include fatty foods and carbohydrate, but also high protein foods and alcohol. Caloric excess is particularly significant when the plasma triglyceride level is already elevated and is less important in the genesis of the hyperlipidemia when only the plasma cholesterol level is increased.

There are two metabolic consequences of excessive calories and adiposity in hypertriglyceridemic patients. With an increased caloric substrate for triglyceride synthesis in the liver, VLDL secretion into the plasma is increased (25). The second consequence is reduced clearance of triglyceride from the plasma. Enlarged adipose tissue cells may have a reduced capacity to remove circulating triglyceride from the plasma, perhaps because of their lessened sensitivity to circulating insulin, which activates lipoprotein lipase. Many hypertriglyceridemic patients have overt diabetes mellitus or abnormal glucose tolerance curves. However, not all mildly or profoundly obese persons have hypertriglyceridemia. Adiposity plus a lipoprotein clearing defect are probably both needed before hypertriglyceridemia results.

Since the typical American adult consumes too much food which contains excessive calories, cholesterol, and saturated fat, in many hypertriglyceridemic patients there is an associated hypercholesterolemia. Of course VLDL carries some cholesterol but LDL may also be increased, since VLDL is its precursor. Moderate reduction of caloric intake in hypertriglyceridemic overweight patients and the subsequent loss of adiposity invariably lead to lower plasma lipid levels, perhaps even to a normal range. Plasma cholesterol levels concomitantly fall (25,26).

While caloric control is the most important consideration for these hypertriglyceridemic patients, the source of the calories in the diets to produce weight loss is of some importance in the establishment of patterns of food consumption that will be useful later when a more ideal weight has been achieved. Many patients with mixed or combined hyperlipidemia (i.e., type II-b) will have some hypercholesterolemia remaining after body weight stabilizes at a more ideal figure. This will require further attention. Furthermore, the pattern of food intake should then be such that future weight gain is avoided. As will be developed subsequently, the single diet or alternative diet concept can be useful for both the period of weight reduction and the subsequent period of body weight stabilization.

Carbohydrates

From all of the evidence available, it should now be emphasized that amount and type of carbohydrate per se consumed in natural diets has had little or no long term effect upon the plasma lipid levels. This statement is contrary to previous thinking that dietary carbohydrate might elevate the plasma triglyceride level. Many of the diets prescribed in the past for the treatment of hypertriglyceridemia laid stress upon a low carbohydrate, high fat diet in which the fat was largely polyunsaturated.

It is true that a sudden increase in the amount of carbohydrate in the diet produces an initial temporary and artificial elevation of plasma triglyceride concentrations, the so-called carbohydrate-induced hyperlipidemia. This short term phenomenon is well established in both normal and hyperlipidemic Americans who have been given high carbohydrate diets (65 to 90% of the total calories). Most of these studies, however, have been of only a few days or at best a few weeks duration. To be emphasized is the fact that populations consuming high carbohydrate diets (up to 80% of total calories in contrast to the usual American intake of 45% of total calories) habitually have a low incidence of atherosclerosis and do not have markedly elevated plasma triglyceride levels (4). In the short term experimental studies in which the dietary carbohydrate has been increased from 45% of total calories, there is usually, but not always, a sharp rise in plasma triglyceride and only a slight increase, if any, in the plasma cholesterol level (27,28). Table 4 depicts the plasma triglyceride responses of six subjects whose baseline diet contained 40% of the total calories from fat, 15% from protein, and 65% from carbohydrate. The plasma triglyceride level rose in all subjects, peaked during the first weeks, and returned to the baseline levels by 4 weeks (28). Longer term studies have indicated that plasma triglyceride concentration may remain elevated for as long as 20 weeks and then subsequently return to the baseline levels (30). The response of normal and diabetic Americans to increased dietary carbohydrate over long periods of time has actually been a lowering of serum lipid levels, provided that dietary cholesterol and fat have been concurrently lowered as described earlier (31,32).

There is no evidence to indicate that a decrease in the usual American intake of dietary carbohydrate (45% of total calories) would be beneficial to patients with hypertriglyceridemia. The evidence that weight reduction and decreased dietary cholesterol and saturated fat result in lower VLDL is overwhelming in comparison to any effect that decreasing dietary carbohydrate might conceivably have upon plasma triglyceride levels. Indeed, patients with hypertriglyceridemia given a high fat diet have delayed clearance of dietary triglyceride absorbed into the body and thus show an intense and additive postprandial hypertriglyceridemia (33). This point is lost sight of when only fasting plasma values are obtained. Conversely, hypertriglyceridemic patients given high carbohydrate meals have a postprandial depression of plasma triglyceride levels (34).

Table 4   The Sequential Plasma Triglyceride Changes from a High Carbohydrate (CHO) Diet (Transitory CHO Induced Hyperlipidemia)

	Basal Diet	High CHO Diet	
	40% Fat	20% Fat	
	45% CHO	65% CHO	
		Plasma Triglyceride (mg/dl)	
		Peak Value during First	
Subject		2 Weeks	4 Weeks
1	60	105	73
2	100	148	94
3	108	224	156
4	131	201	145
5	160	215	142
6	197	224	213
Mean ± SD	126 ± 48	186 ± 49	137 ± 49
Significance (paired t test)		$p < 0.005^a$	$p < 0.005^b$

[a] Compared to 126 ± 48.
[b] Compared to 186 ± 49.

The Kind of Dietary Carbohydrate

The metabolic response in man to the ingestion of dietary carbohydrate has been felt by some investigators to depend on the type of carbohydrate given. In the 1960s, it was suggested that the high sucrose consumption of the European-American populations might have an important role in the pathogenesis of coronary heart disease (35). The basis of this hypothesis related almost entirely to an association between the amount of sucrose consumed in the diet by various population groups and the mortality from coronary heart disease. However, considerable uncertainty has developed about the validity of this hypothesis. Atherosclerosis readily produced in experimental animals by cholesterol feeding has not occurred in animals simply fed sucrose. For example, the rhesus monkey fed a cholesterol-free, low fat diet with 40% of the calories from sucrose for 3 years did not develop either atherosclerosis or hyperlipidemia (6). This would seem a convincing experiment about the general nonatherogenecity of dietary sucrose per se.

The initial observations about the hyperlipidemic effects of dietary sucrose in man (36) have not been verified by later investigation, particularly if caloric balance was carefully controlled (28,37,38). In addition, in all of these studies, the amounts of sucrose fed were much greater than Americans ordinarily eat. A study of the interrelationship between the kinds of dietary carbohydrate in hyperlipoproteinemic subjects has indicated that sucrose generally has not elevated plasma lipid levels over levels of a control starch period (28,39).

This being said, we then come to the pratical conclusion that it seems sound to recommend a moderate decrease in the consumption of sucrose and other simple sugars for most hyperlipidemic patients who are overweight. Sugar constitutes a highly concentrated source of calories, which is eaten for pleasure in large quantities. It is a contributor to the problem of obesity, and to dental caries as well. In addition, sucrose, like fat and alcohol, provides only empty calories in the sense that it does not contain associated protein, fiber, minerals, and vitamins as do other unrefined foodstuffs (cereals, legumes, fruits, and vegetables). The treatment of hyperlipidemia may require the correction of excessive adiposity, which can only be accomplished by a great decrease in total caloric intake, of which sugar is usually such a large component in the typical American diet. The bulk content of the diet (i.e., fiber) is also increased.

Fiber

Dietary fiber is a nondescript term which includes several carbohydrates thought to be indigestible by the human gut. These are cellulose, hemicellulose, lignin, and pectin. Dietary fiber is commonly found in cereals, legumes, vegetables, and fruits. In ruminant animals, dietary fiber is completely digested by the microbial flora of the rumen, so that fiber provides a major source of energy for these animals. In man, however, dietary fiber contributes considerable bulk to the diet, but from evidence to date, probably contributes little to the caloric content of the diet.

Fiber experiments date back at least 20 years. Plasma lipid lowering effects greater than might be expected from changes in dietary fat and cholesterol were earlier reported by Keys and co-workers from the feeding of legumes and pectins (40,41). Fiber added to semisynthetic diets fed to rats has usually resulted in lower levels of plasma cholesterol. In man, however, the literature on fiber feeding provides little evidence that most dietary fibers contained in natural foods are hypocholesterolemic per se (42). However, when two sources of fiber, pectin or guar gum, are taken as pharmaceutical agents, some plasma cholesterol lowering is achieved.

Diets which are low in cholesterol and saturated fat and which are high in complex carbohydrates derived from partially unrefined food-stuffs are automatically high in fiber content. The fiber content of these diets (up to 18 mg/day) is similar to that of the diets of primitive man and also to that of the diets of most of the nonaffluent populations of the world (34,44,45). It is worth noting that the peoples mentioned above have low levels of serum lipids and a low incidence of coronary heart disease (43,44). Thus, a diet naturally high in fiber is easy to devise and consume. The probable major importance of dietary fiber in hyperlipidemic states is indirect. In the customary American diet, foods high in fiber have been replaced with foods of high caloric density, which also have a high cholesterol and saturated fat content. When these foods are replaced by foods naturally high in dietary fiber, the intake of cholesterol and saturated fat usually decreases concomitantly.

Alcohol

Alcohol ingestion has a variable effect upon the plasma lipid levels which is related to the dose and duration of ingestion. Insignificant increases in serum cholesterol levels occur as a result of alcohol ingestion. However, the plasma triglyceride may increase in normal or alcoholic subjects given large amounts of alcohol (up to 8 to 10 ounces/day of whiskey or the equivalent) (46–48). These effects are frequently transient. Often the period of alcohol feeding has also been hypercaloric, so that the effects of alcohol upon the serum lipids may well result from the caloric content of the added alcohol alone.

Certain people are very sensitive to caloric excess supplied as alcohol and respond by a prompt increase in plasma VLDL and triglyceride. Other foodstuffs in hypercaloric additions might well have had the same elevating effects on serum lipid. The mechanisms whereby alcohol might affect the serum lipid levels include the impairment of plasma triglyceride removal and increased synthesis of triglyceride-rich lipoproteins (49).

As a source of additional calories, alcohol could clearly contribute to caloric excess, to obesity, and, in some individuals, to hyperlipidemia for that reason. The consumption of calories from alcohol may be an important consideration in the overweight, hypertriglyceridemic patient. The usual single drink—whiskey, gin, beer, or wine—contains about 140 calories. Four drinks per day would thus contribute 560 calories, or one-fifth to one-fourth of the total caloric needs of most individuals. During the period of weight reduction, alcohol is best avoided altogether. When ideal weight has been obtained, small quantities of alcohol may be instituted to note whether hypertriglyceridemia occurs or is accentuated. The designated quantities of alcohol must be computed as a part of the total caloric intake. Most patients can consume 1 to 3 ounces of alcohol as part of their total diet and avoid hyperlipidemia, provided weight gain is avoided. However, if such a trial of alcohol produces hyperlipidemia, then its use should be completely discontinued. The use of alcohol is clearly precluded in types I and V patients who have had pancreatitis. Should liver disease and hyperlipidemia occur together, alcohol should not be used under any circumstances.

Protein

Dietary protein has been studied extensively for possible effects on plasma lipid concentrations. These studies have utilized both single protein sources and mixtures of different protein, with ranges of protein intake from 25 to 150 g/day. No changes in the plasma cholesterol and triglyceride concentrations have occurred from these different amounts of protein, provided that at least the minimum amounts of essential amino acids have been ingested. The protein consumed in mixed human diets has not been shown to have significant effects upon plasma lipoprotein and lipid levels in man. For example, egg albumin and casein have been extensively used over the past 20 years in cholesterol-free formula diets which have produced a maximum fall in plasma cholesterol concentrations. When an animal-derived protein, such as casein, has been provided in a semisynthetic diet to an experimental animal like the rabbit, which has such a different lipoprotein transport system and metabolism from man the results can certainly not be extrapolated to the human condition.

In view of the negative results of many experiments involving possible hypercholesterolemic effects of casein, there is currently no reason to think of soybean protein as having unique hypolipidemic characteristics. Future experiments may delineate such an effect. A diet in which animal protein sources, such as meat and eggs, are reduced in quantities not only has vegetable protein replacing animal protein, but also has a reduction in dietary cholesterol and saturated fat. Such a dietary change would be hypolipidemic for reasons already discussed. The alternative diet does make extensive use of proteins from vegetable sources in order to supply the body's needs for sufficient protein.

Lecithin

The lecithin derived from soybeans is a mixture of several phospholipids. Commonly sold in health food stores, it is publicized as a popular remedy for hypercholesterolemia. Aside from its high content of linoleic acid, lecithin has little or no effect upon lipid metabolism. Contrary to popular belief, lecithin is not absorbed as such from the digestive tract but is hydrolized into its constituent fatty acids and choline. Choline is a lipotrophic substance which was tested in the treatment of hypercholesterolemia 25 years ago and found to be of no value. The plasma lecithin levels have not been affected by the addition of lecithin in the diet; the circulating plasma lecithin is largely synthesized by the liver. Parenthetically, high levels of plasma phospholipids are seen in patients with complete biliary obstruction and also in the hypercholesterolemia of the type II-a patient. If one desires to use a high content of linoleic acid in the diet, this can be obtained much more inexpensively from a liquid polyunsaturated vegetable oil.

Minerals and Vitamins

If the minimal daily requirements for minerals and vitamins have been met in the diet, there is no evidence that additional vitamins and minerals will have any effect upon the plasma lipid concentrations. This comment applies equally to vitamin C and vitamin E, again popularly consumed by the public without there being any proof of benefit. Excessive amounts of vitamin D cause hypercalcemia and hence would promote atherogenesis. The one exception is niacin, vitamin B_2, which, when given as a drug in a dose fifty times its requirements as a vitamin, does have a hypolipidemic effect. In this instance, niacin is used as a pharmaceutical preparation and not as a nutrient.

THE IMPLEMENTATION OF THE SINGLE DIET CONCEPT FOR THE TREATMENT OF HYPERLIPIDEMIA

Instead of multiple diets, each for a different form of hyperlipidemia, a single diet concept for the treatment of hyperlipidemia has been evolved into a practical, workable format as a result of newer experimental evidence and clinical trial, as has been previously discussed (Tables 5,6). The chemical formulation of the single diet, termed the Alternative Diet is presented in terms of major components as follows. The ultimate and optimal objectives in terms of a diet to produce maximal lowering of

Table 5 Dietary Factors in the Causation and Correction of Lipoprotein Abnormalities

Lipoprotein Increased	Cause	Dietary Factor Increasing Lipoprotein Synthesis	Dietary Correction
Chylomicrons (types I, V)	Impaired removal	Fat, regardless of relative saturation	Reduction of dietary fat to 5 to 10% of total calories[a]
VLDL (types IV, II-b) and IDL (type III)	Impaired removal (obesity) or increased synthesis or both	Excessive calories from any source Dietary cholesterol and saturated fat	A hypocaloric, 20% fat diet to induce the loss of excess adiposity; reduction of dietary cholestrol and saturated fat
LDL (types II-a, II-b)	Increased synthesis and impaired removal	Dietary cholesterol, saturated fat, and total fat.	Reduction of dietary cholesterol to 100 mg, saturated fat to 5% of total calories, and total fat to 20%.
Lipoprotein decreased HDL	Utilization of HDL apoproteins in triglyceride-carrying lipoproteins in types I, V, II-b, and III hyperlipidemia	Excessive calories with adiposity	Correction of obesity as noted above.

[a] All overweight hyperlipidemic patients should have the appropriate dietary factor modified as above and, in addition, should be provided with a hypocaloric diet to help in the attainment of normal body weight. Likewise, if the patient is an insulin-dependent diabetic, appropriate use of insulin may also aid in the correction of the hyperlipidemia.

Table 6   Nutrient Composition of the Present American Diet and the "Alternative Diet"[a]

	American Diet	Alternative Diet (Phase III)
Cholesterol (mg/day)	750	100
Fat (% of total calories)	40	20
Saturated fat (% calories)	15	5
Monounsaturated fat (% calories)	16	8
Polyunsaturated fat (% calories)	6	7
P/S value	0.4	1.3
Iodine number	63	99
Vegetable fat (% fat)	38	75
Animal fat (% fat)	62	25
Protein (% calories)	15	15
Vegetable protein (% protein)	32	56
Animal protein (% protein)	68	44
Carbohydrate (% calories)	45	65
Starch (% calories)	22	40
Sucrose (added to food) (% calories)	15	10
Fructose, glucose, sucrose, lactose, maltose (% calories) (naturally present in foods)	8	15
Crude fiber (g)	2–3	12–15
Sodium (mEq)	200–300	50–75[a]
Potassium (mEq)	30–70	120–150

[a] Should sodium restriction be necessary.

plasma lipid will be achieved in a series of phases to be described in detail with appropriate menu planning and recipes.

Dietary Cholesterol

Dietary cholesterol is reduced from the usual American intake of 600 to 800 mg/day to 100 mg/day. This change will lower LDL cholesterol, which is elevated in types II-a and II-b hyperlipidemia, and also both VLDL and intermediate density lipoprotein (IDL) in types IV and III hyperlipidemias, respectively (Table 5). In many patients with diet-induced II-a or II-b hypercholesterolemia, a reduction of dietary cholesterol to 100 mg/day will lower the plasma lipids to normal values (plasma cholesterol level below 220 mg/dl). Frequently, hyperlipidemic patients are also overweight. For overweight patients, the same diet, at a hypocaloric level, should be prescribed initially until the patient attains optimum weight. At that point, the Alternative Diet at a eucaloric level is prescribed.

Endogenous type II-a (severe) hypercholesterolemia is genetically derived, with dietary factors having only an additive role in these patients. Although normal plasma cholesterol levels cannot usually be achieved by dietary measures alone, nevertheless, a diet in conjunction at times with drugs has assumed an important aspect in the treatment of familial hypercholesterolemia. Dietary cholesterol restriction is even more important in the severe type II-a patient.

Total Dietary Fat

The dietary fat content is lowered to 20% of total calories compared with the usual American fat intake of 40% of calories. Most of the fat reduction is saturated or hard fat, with the saturated fat content maintained at no more than 5% of total calories. This change in total content and composition has a beneficial effect in all forms of hyperlipidemia for reasons already discussed but especially in type II and types I and V hyperlipidemia (Table 5). Patients with types I and V hyperlipidemia have extreme hypertriglyceridemia largely because of the delayed clearance of absorbed dietary fat. When dietary fat is reduced to a minimum, the chylomicrons present in the blood gradually clear and the plasma triglycerides fall. Plasma cholesterol levels also decline. This minimum of dietary fat varies from patient to patient; the exact level necessary for chylomicron clearance will be ascertained only by the trial of several diets of differing fat content. In some patients the 20% fat diet may be appropriate. In other patients the lowest possible fat content—a diet that contains only 5 to 10% of the calories as fat—may be essential. Such a diet does provide over 1% of the total calories as linoleic acid to meet essential fatty acid requirements. To enhance its palatability, a small quantity of medium-chain triglycerides (MCT^R) can be incorporated into the diet. In some patients with extreme chylomicronemia who are in danger of acute pancreatitis, a fat-free formula diet (protein, glucose, minerals, and vitamins) can be employed to promote maximal chylomicron lowering. Another simple but effective approach would be the use of fruit juices for a few days of initial therapy. Restriction of calories if the patient is overweight can be carried out simultaneously.

In a few days, triglyceride levels may fall from over 6000 mg/dl to below 1000 to 2000 mg/dl.

There is a great danger in treating a hypertriglyceridemic subject with a high fat, low carbohydrate diet if the patient has fasting chylomicronemia. Such was the case for an 18-month-old infant, profoundly hypertriglyceridemic, who had been treated for several months with the high fat, low CHO, type IV diet which contained 45% of the calories from fat. This patient continued to have elevated plasma triglyceride levels and recurrent attacks of abdominal pain, and even pancreatitis, in spite of what was apparently an appropriate diet. This patient was actually misdiagnosed as a type IV patient and was therefore given a high fat diet, with an exacerbation of symptoms as a result. Table 7 shows his plasma triglyceride response to a very low fat diet (5% of the calories). Another patient, a 26-year-old adult with profound hypertriglyceridemia, was given a high fat, polyunsaturated diet in a therapeutic effort to control his hyperlipidemia. One month later he developed acute hemorrhagic pancreatitis with plasma triglyceride concentrations of over 7000 mg/dl. This patient was subsequently diagnosed as having type V hyperlipidemia and was treated with the very low fat diet. The plasma triglyceride level fell to under 800 mg/dl, largely as VLDL with no fasting chylomicrons. Subsequent episodes of pancreatitis were avoided.

With the use of the single diet concept for the treatment of hyperlipidemia, these type I and type V patients with hyperchylomicronemia, if the problem was critical, would initially be given a very low fat diet (5 to 10% of the total calories) with 75 to 80% of the calories as carbohydrate. As fasting chylomicronemia improved to a plasma triglyceride level of below 1000 mg/dl, the next step would be to increase the

Table 7   Plasma Triglyceride Response to a Low Fat Diet in a Patient with Profound Hypertriglyceridemia and Chylomicronemia

Diet	Plasma Triglycerides (mg/dl)
"Type IV diet," 45% fat, 36% CHO	5340
Low fat diet, 5% fat, 70 to 75% CHO	
After 4 days	1860
After 8 days	807

dietary fat to 15 to 20% of the total calories in order to judge the tolerance to dietary fat.

While the basic problem in types I and V hyperlipidemia is not an excess of dietary cholesterol, and the suggested diets do not restrict cholesterol per se, they are lower in cholesterol content because most foods containing cholesterol are also high in fat. However, shellfish, which are relatively high in cholesterol content, are low in fat content and in saturated fat. Consequently, they can be used freely by patients with types I and V hyperlipidemia.

Saturated Fat

The saturated fat content of the diet is reduced to promote the lowering of LDL in types II-a and II-b. This change, in conjunction with the restriction of dietary cholesterol, will produce a maximal lowering of LDL and the plasma cholesterol concentration. The polyunsaturated fat content remains little changed from the usual American intake of 6 to 8% of total calories for reasons that have been discussed previously. Because the saturated fat content is decreased, the P/S value of the dietary fat increases from 0.4 to 1.3. Most of the reduction of the total fat from 40% of the total calories to 20% is accomplished by cutting down foods that are rich in saturated fatty acid content.

Because the fat content of the diet is reduced and the protein intake is kept at an amount similar to what Americans commonly eat, namely, about 15% of the total calories, the carbohydrate content of the diet must be increased.The decrease in fat is thus offset by a reciprocal increase in dietary carbohydrate. Ultimately, the amount of dietary carbohydrate will be 65% of the total calories, with the increased amount of carbohydrate being provided for in terms of complex carbohydrate ordinarily associated with protein as well. Other constituents of the diet are not reduced or even enhanced in terms of nutritional adequacy, as will be discussed subsequently.

Caloric Control

Caloric control is vitally important in overweight patients for decreasing the VLDL of types II-b and IV and the IDL of type III hyperlipidemia and in improving the chylomicron clearance for type V hyperlipidemia (Table 5). The plasma triglyceride response to caloric restriction and weight loss is usually prompt and dramatic in types IV and II-b patients. The lowered triglyceride level is sustained as long as weight loss continues. With the achievement of normal weight, the plasma triglyceride level usually remains in the normal range. Glucose intolerance and the associated diabetic state may also disappear with the hypertriglyceridemia.

The special case of the overweight type II-b patient warrants further comment. After the excessive plasma triglyceride levels are corrected by weight loss, this patient may be left with some hypercholesterolemia carried by LDL. Particular attention will need to be directed to the restriction of dietary cholesterol and fat when the eucaloric diet to maintain weight is initiated.

To use the Alternative Diet in the correction of obesity, the caloric prescription should be cut in half or below if the patient is overweight. Thus, an individual whose caloric requirements are estimated to be 2400 calories should have a dietary prescription of the Alternative Diet in any of the particular phases of 1000 to 1200 calories.

A PHASED ALTERNATIVE DIET APPROACH TO THE TREATMENT OF HYPERLIPIDEMIA

A realistic view is that even well-motivated patients have difficulties in making abrupt changes in their dietary habits. It may take many months or even a year to change food consumption patterns. Therefore, the changes recommended from the current American diet of most hyperlipidemic patients should be approached in a gradual manner, with each of three phases introducing more changes toward the alternative dietary pattern ultimately required for maximal therapy (3,50).

Phase I

The goal of phase I is to modify the customary consumption of foods very high in cholesterol and saturated fat. This can be accomplished by deleting egg yolk, butterfat, lard, and organ meats from the diet and by using substitute products when possible: soft margarine for butter, vegetable oils and shortening for lard, skim milk and egg whites for whole eggs. Many alternative foods to replace foods that contain large amounts of cholesterol and saturated fat are now marketed (50).

Many recipes currently in use can be modified with the retention of their usual tastiness. For example, most recipes, including baked items, can be made without egg yolks. Usually 1½ to 2 egg whites can be used successfully in place of 1 whole egg. This modification has been used in making cakes, cookies, custards (adding yellow food color), potato salad, and many other products without changing the quality. Many recipes can also be altered to use less fat and to use vegetable oils instead of animal fat.

Summary of Phase I

Avoid foods very high in cholesterol and saturated fat. Delete egg yolk, butterfat, lard, and organ meats. Substitute soft margarine for butter; vegetable oils and shortening for lard; skim milk for whole milk; egg whites for whole eggs.

Phase II

In phase II, a reduction of meat consumption is the goal, with a gradual transition from the American ideal of up to a pound of meat a day to no more than 6 to 8 ounces per day. Meat can no longer occupy the center of the meal, particularly for two or three meals each day. One significant point is the change in the composition of the traditional sandwich. Meat and cheese are not necessarily essential parts of a sandwich, nor is a sandwich always necessary for lunch. In addition, in phase II, we propose the use of less fat and cheese.

At this time, new recipes are needed to replace the recipes that cannot be altered to meet this new way of eating (50). Substitute recipes have been developed to replace recipes in which meat or high fat dairy products (cream cheese, butter, sour cream, cheese) are the principal ingredients. Since these foods are to be used in smaller amounts or even omitted, the patient must use recipes that include larger amounts of grains, legumes, vegetables and fruits. Furthermore, because of the worldwide concern for the conservation of natural resources and the use of economical foods, as well as to tap the current interest in gourmet cooking and exotic foods, a large number of new recipes can be found in current cookbooks, magazines, and newspapers. Many of these stress the use of nonanimal food products. With these new ways of eating, the diet will employ a wide variety of spices and different products and foods from the cuisines of other countries. Many cultures have developed delicious meals which are low in cholesterol and low in fat. Oriental dishes emphasize fresh vegetables and rice products; Mexican dishes lay stress on various tortillas, peppers, and beans. The Mediterranean countries (Greece, Italy, and Spain) incorporate pastas and vegetable sauces in meals. The cuisine of the Middle Eastern countries employs a variety of wheat products and legume dishes. These are only a few of the available examples.

Summary of Phase II

Gradually decrease meat consumption from up to 16 ounces a day to no more than 6 to 8 ounces once a day. Use less fat and cheese. Acquire new recipes.

Phase III

In phase III, the maximal diet for the treatment of hyperlipidemia is attained. The cholesterol content of the diet is reduced to 100 mg/day and the saturated fat is lowered to 5 to 6% of the total calories. These changes mean that meat consumption, in particular, must be further reduced. For most patients, this will present a problem of considerable magnitude. In order to deal with this problem we take an historical approach to the consumption of meat. Man has always eaten meat. What he has not done is to eat meat every day, let alone several times a day. Even today, daily meat consumption is possible only for the affluent minority of the world's population, since it is a very costly food in terms of the utilization of natural resources.

In phase III, meat, fish, and poultry should be used as "condiments" rather than "aliments." With this philosophy, no longer will the meat dish occupy the center of the table. Instead, meat in smaller quantities will spice up vegetable-rice-cereal-legume-based dishes, much as Oriental, Indian, and Mediterranean cookery has been doing for generations. The use of special low cholesterol cheeses is also an important component of phase III.

The total of meat, fish, and poultry should average 3 to 4 ounces/ day, but the use of fish and poultry should be stressed because of their lower saturated fat content. By this time, the new recipes will be emphasizing whole grains and legumes. In phase III of the Alternative Diet, lunch, the smaller meal of the day, is changed by using beans, grains, and low fat animal products in place of meat. The larger meal of the day, dinner, should be altered particularly in phase III. A large variety of new flavors and spices will be introduced. An example of entrees for dinner over a week include beef or pork for 2 days, poultry for 2 days, fish for 2 days, and meatless for 1 day.

Eating Away From Home and Entertainment on Special Occasions

Many restaurants serve a wide variety of the foods recommended in the different phases of the Alternative Diet. The cuisine of Oriental, Italian,

Mexican, and Middle Eastern restaurants all have tasty foods to choose from. In the inevitable situation where food choices are minimal, such as at parties or when eating in friends' homes, one can concentrate on the salad, vegetable, fruit, and cereal foods and take only small amounts of the animal foods. Guests entertained at home can be introduced to a new way of eating which they will discover to be attractive, tasty, and healthful. Certain foods should be saved for special occasions or feast days: extra meat, shellfish, regular cheese, chocolate, candy, and coconut. During phase III, the transition from the current American diet to the Alternative Diet will be completed to provide for the maximal treatment of the hyperlipidemic state.

Summary of Phase III

Eat mainly cereals, legumes, fruits and vegetables. Use meat as a condiment. Use low cholesterol cheeses. Save these foods for use only on special occasions: extra meats, regular cheeses, chocolate, candy, and coconut.

A Food Guide for the Alternative Diet is depicted in Figure 5. The

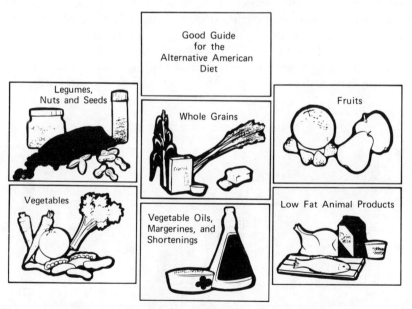

Figure 5. Six food groups representing the Alternative Diet. Emphasis is placed on the consumption of whole grains, legumes, vegetables, and fruits. Only one of the six food groups contains low fat animal products, contrasted to the four food groups in the current American diet in which two of four food groups contain animal products.

dietary plan emphasizes six food groups: whole grains; legumes, nuts, and seeds; vegetables; fruits; vegetable oils, margarine, and shortenings; and low fat animal products. A variety of foods from each of these six food groups should be consumed each day. The majority of food intake will be derived from grains, grain products, potatoes, legumes, fruits, and vegetables. Low fat animal products (skim milk, egg whites, low fat cheeses, etc.) and substitutes for animal products should be included. Meat and added vegetable fat are to be used as condiments.

THE CHEMICAL COMPOSITION OF THE ALTERNATIVE DIET

The chemical composition of the American diet as well as of the three phases of the Alternative Diet is given in Figure 6. The American diet contains approximately 600 to 700 mg of cholesterol per day. This is decreased in phase I to 450 mg, in phase II to 300 mg, and in phase III to 100 mg/day. The fat content decreases from 40% of calories in the American diet, to 35% in phase I, to 25% in phase II, and to 20% in phase III with special consideration given to the decrease of saturated fat. In order to have sufficient calories to meet body needs, the carbohydrate content should be increased as the fat content is decreased, with emphasis on the use of the fiber-containing complex carbohydrates contained in whole grains, cereal products, and legumes. The carbohydrate content increases from 45% of calories in the American diet,

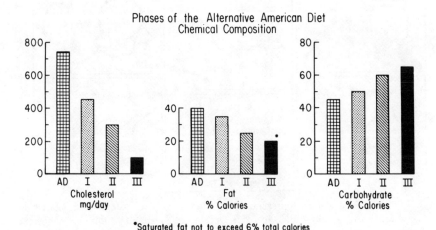

*Saturated fat not to exceed 6% total calories

Figure 6. The cholesterol, fat, and carbohydrate content of the American diet (AD) and the phases (I, II, III) of the Alternative Diet.

to 50% in phase I, to 60% in phase II, and to 65% in phase III. This increases the bulk of the diets considerably, a feature which induces satiety sooner per unit of calories and helps to promote weight loss. The crude fiber content in the Alternative Diet increases from 4 gm/day to 12 g/day.

PREDICTED PLASMA CHOLESTEROL LOWERING FROM THE THREE PHASES OF THE ALTERNATIVE DIET

As has been emphasized, both dietary cholesterol and saturated fat elevate plasma cholesterol levels, whereas polyunsaturated fat has a mild depressing effect. In stepwise fashion, the cholesterol and saturated fat of each phase of the Alternative Diet are successively reduced, with phase III providing for the lowest intakes. According to calculations derived from Hegsted and co-workers (20), phase III of the Alternative Diet would lower maximal plasma cholesterol levels by an estimated 77 mg/dl. Phase II would produce a lowering of 49 mg/dl, and phase I, 28 mg/dl. These plasma cholesterol changes for all phases offer the possibilities of improved plasma lipids, dependent upon the amount of dietary modification, phase III being the ultimate goal.

THE RESPONSE TO TREATMENT IN OUTPATIENTS FROM THE USE OF THE ALTERNATIVE DIET

The 100 mg low cholesterol Alternative Diet (phase III) was followed by 96 outpatients with various forms of hyperlipidemia and xanthomatosis, and some with diabetes mellitus. The composite results in the mixed group of hyperlipidemic individuals with types II-a, II-b, III, and IV are shown in Figure 7. The plasma cholesterol concentrations declined tremendously, some 94mg/dl, or a decrease of 30% over 2 years. There was also a decrease in the plasma triglyceride concentrations. There were no type I or V patients in this treatment group. They would, of course, have required, in most instances, further restriction of dietary fat down to 10% of the total calories.

THE USE OF THE ALTERNATIVE DIET IN DIABETES AND PREGNANCY

The approach to the diabetic patient who is also hyperlipidemic involves the same dietary considerations as for the treatment of the hyperlipi-

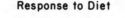

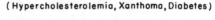

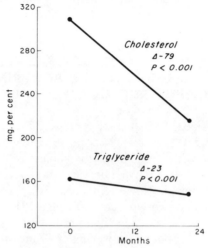

Figure 7.   The use of the phase III, 100 mg cholesterol, low fat diet in 96 hyperlipidemic outpatients followed for 24 months.

demia. Phase III of the Alternative Diet has been used successfully in both juvenile-onset and maturity-onset diabetic patients, both insulin dependent and noninsulin dependent (31). Clearly involved in this treatment is the appropriate control of carbohydrate as well as lipid metabolism by the adequate amounts of insulin and weight reduction when the patient is overweight. The great propensity of diabetic patients to atherosclerotic vascular disease makes control of their hyperlipidemia of particular importance. The principles outlined as above can be utilized fully with benefit to the patient.

Pregnancy constitutes a particularly difficult situation because in most pregnant women there will be some 40 to 50% increase in plasma lipids and lipoproteins (chiefly LDL) under physiological circumstances. The hyperlipidemic patient who becomes pregnant should clearly continue on the same diet advised previously for the treatment of her hyperlipidemia. As already stressed, this diet is nutritionally adequate. The pregnant hyperlipidemic patient would receive the same supplemental minerals and vitamins as the usual patient during pregnancy.

Circumstances that these authors have repeatedly been called upon to deal with include the patient with familial hypercholesterolemia (type II-a) who becomes pregnant, and also the type I or V patient who becomes pregnant. In the former instance, the 100 mg low cholesterol, 20% fat, phase III of the Alternative Diet is utilized with some increase in calories to permit the desired weight gain. In the type I and V hypertriglyceridemic pregnant patient, there is apt to be a profound augmentation of the usual hyperchylomicronemia and delay in clearance of plasma triglyceride. Again, stricter adherence to the low fat 5 to 10% diet is cautioned.

THE SINGLE DIET FOR THE TREATMENT OF HYPERLIPIDEMIC CHILDREN

The single diet concept for the treatment of hyperlipidemic children can be applied as for adults. Egg yolk, organ meat, and butterfat are eliminated from the diet, even for infants. Dietary iron is supplemented from fortified cereals. Human breast milk, or whole cow's milk, is recommended prior to weaning or until the infant eats sufficient table food to provide adequate calories for growth. This is usually from 1 to 2 years. From that time on, the infant should drink skim milk.

This is not a drastic alteration in the way infants are currently being fed. Since World War II, a large number of American babies have been, and continue to be, fed commercially prepared formulas which are low in cholesterol and reduced in saturated fat content. The American infant is given a cholesterol-free milk-based formula and then later, during or after weaning, is given foods with high concentrations of cholesterol such as egg yolk, liver, and strained meats. We propose a reversal of this procedure. Initially, infants should receive whole milk and later not be given solid foods high in cholesterol content. This would provide for a sufficient quantity of exogenous cholesterol which conceivably may be needed during the immediate postnatal period of rapid growth and development. In addition, this proposed dietary plan decreases the large quantity of polyunsaturated fat and plant sterols the infants receive from artificial formulas. Plant sterols have been found in the plasma and tissues of infants receiving these vegetable oil, cholesterol-free formulas and their long term effects are completely unknown (51). With maturity of the gastrointestinal tract, the plant sterols of the diet are presumably not absorbed as they must be in early infancy.

The use of the maximal plasma cholesterol lowering diet is most critical for the most common form of hyperlipidemia in children, familial hypercholesterolemia (type II-a). Even in the homozygous hyper-cholesterolemic child, a decrease in plasma cholesterol will occur with the Alternative Diet with its dietary restriction of 100 mg/day or less,

Our experience with two homozygous children is illustrative. Di, age 16, had an initial plasma cholesterol of 664 ± 28 mg/dl; her sister, De, age 13, had 776 ± 54 mg/dl. After only dietary treatment, the plasma cholesterol of Di was 519 ± 13 and that of De, 604 ± 47 mg/dl, decreases of 145 and 162 mg/dl, and −22 and −21% respectively.

For the rare infant with type I hyperlipidemia, the fat content of the usual human breast or cow's milk will need to be cut down. A basic skim milk formula will need to be used to avoid the abdominal pain and episodes of pancreatitis that these patients so often experience. The main objective of such therapy is the provision of sufficient amounts of essential fatty acid which can be prescribed separately as safflower or sunflower seed oil to yield at least 1 to 2% of the total calories. In this way, most of the fat intake will be from linoleic acid and very little other fat will be taken in. Success in several infants with type I disorder has been achieved using this dietary approach, with the abolition of episodes of abdominal pain.

THE USE OF THE ALTERNATIVE DIET BY THE FAMILY

In most instances hyperlipidemia and coronary heart disease are familial diseases, both because of genetic predisposition and because of the nutrition imbalances that usually develop in the family setting. Thus, the treatment by diet of one family member with hyperlipidemia usually means that other family members should likewise be identified and treated. This is important because it is difficult to initiate dietary change in a single member of the family because food is consumed largely in the family group. The preparation of several different menus is both difficult and irksome. As already mentioned, children especially should be included in this consideration for possible familial treatment. First, atherosclerosis is a continuously progressive process throughout life which has its beginnings in childhood. Second, food consumption patterns are learned early in life.

The age of the patient in the life situation in which treatment is initiated is of utmost importance. If the propositus is a child, then his parents as well as his older and younger siblings may be hyperlipidemic. If the propositus is an adult, then other family members may well have the problem, including children. The use of the Alternative Diet for the entire family is certainly suggested. The diet is nutritionally adequate for all family members and since hyperlipidemia is a family problem, most individuals in the family would benefit. None would be harmed.

β-SITOSTEROLEMIA AND XANTHOMATOSIS, A PLANT STEROL STORAGE DISEASE

A rare familial disease was recently described in two sisters and has been verified now in six other patients (2). It is characterized by the accumulation of plant sterols, particularly β-sitosterol, in the blood and tissues. The prominent clinical manifestations of the disease reported to date are xanthomas of tendons and skin appearing in childhood despite normal or only slightly elevated plasma cholesterol concentration. The plasma plant sterols are greatly increased and the tissues contain large concentrations of plant sterols. Plant sterols are normally absent, or are present in only trace amounts in the body.

The metabolic defects causing the disease are twofold: greatly increased intestinal absorption of dietary β-sitosterol and other plant sterols which are normally absorbed only in minute amounts, and impaired excretion of β-sitosterol from the body. The exact nature of these metabolic defects is unknown. The disease appears to be inherited as an autosomal recessive trait.

The three plant sterols, β-sitosterol, campesterol, and stigmasterol, are usually found only in the lipids of plants, and thus are particularly plentiful in vegetable oils, nuts, and fat-rich vegetables and fruits. In chemical structure, the three plant sterols resemble cholesterol except for minor differences in their side chains.

In normal humans, the intestinal absorption of plant sterols is limited to less than 5% of the amount in the diet. Thus, these sterols pass directly through the intestinal tract and are usually recovered quantitatively in the feces. Twenty per cent of what dietary β-sitosterol is absorbed is converted to bile acids and the remainder is excreted in the bile as the free sterol. Normally, only minute amounts of plant sterols are detectable in the blood of humans. The plasma concentration of β-sitosterol ranges from 0.3 to 1.73 mg/100 ml in humans consuming the typical American diet. However, during infancy, considerable amounts of β-sitosterol can be found in the blood (up to 9 mg/100 ml) and also in the aortas of infants fed vegetable oil-rich formulas (51). In large quantities, plant sterols inhibit cholesterol absorption. A drug rich in plant sterols, Cytellin[R], has long been used to treat hypercholesterolemia.

Laboratory Abnormalities

High concentrations of β-sitosterol and the other two plant sterols in the plasma are the chief characteristics of β-sitosterolemia and xanthomatosis. From 18 to 37 mg/100 ml and from 7 to 16% of the total plasma sterols are plant sterols. The β-sitosterol predominates in concentrations ranging between 12 to 27 mg/100 ml. The campesterol concentration is 6 to 10 mg/100 ml, while less than 1 mg/100 ml of stigmasterol is present. About 60% of the plasma β-sitosterol and campesterol is esterified.

Considerable accumulation of plant sterols occurs in the tendon xanthomas. As in the plasma, β-sitosterol is the most plentiful sterol. The plant sterols present in tendon xanthomas are primarily unesterified. Despite the high content of plant sterols, cholesterol is still the predominant sterol, constituting 73 to 88% of the total sterols. Histologically, these xanthomatous lesions are indistinguishable from the tendon xanthomas found in hyperlipoproteinemia and in cerebrotendonous xanthomatosis.

Dietary Treatment

The logical treatment of this sterol storage disease is a diet low in or devoid of plant sterols, since the excessive plant sterols in the body originate from the diet. Such treatment has reduced the plasma plant sterols but not to the very low levels found normally. Presumably the great stores of plant sterols in the tissues are in equilibration with plant sterols of plasma, and prolonged dietary treatment would be required to reduce the plasma β-sitosterol level to normal.

The guiding principles in the formulation of a diet low in plant sterol content are (1) to eliminate all sources of vegetable fats such as vegetable oil, shortenings, and margarines; (2) to eliminate all plant foods with high fat content such as nuts, seeds, chocolate, olives, and avocado; and (3) to use only refined cereal products which have the germ (rich in fat and plant sterols) removed. In general, foods that have a high content of vegetable fat will also have a high plant sterol content. This therapeutic diet contains most fruits and vegetables, refined cereal products (bread, made with lard or fat free, rice, macaroni, and spaghetti), and foods derived from animal sources which contain cholesterol as the characteristic sterol. These would include meat and meat products, butter and lard, cheese, eggs, milk, and cream. Fish and certain shellfish (shrimp and lobster) may also be eaten as components of the diet low in plant sterols. However, clams, scallops, oysters, and some species of crab must be avoided because they contain sterols which resemble the plant sterols (such as 24-methylene cholesterol and brassicasterol) in amounts up to 50% of the total sterols. These sterols may be absorbed by the intestine like plant sterols and could contribute to the pathogenesis of the disease.

A diet very low in plant sterols is thus, in some respects, diametrically opposite to the low cholesterol diet used in the treatment of hypercholesterolemia.

REFERENCES

1. W. E. Connor, *Biochemistry of Atherosclerosis*, Marcel Dekker, New York, (in press, 1978).
2. A. K. Bhattacharyya and W. E. Connor, *The Metabolic Basis of Inherited Disease*, 4th Ed., McGraw-Hill, New York, 1978, p. 648.
3. W. E. Connor and S. L. Connor, *Hyperlipidemia: Diagnosis and Therapy*, Grune and Stratton, New York, 1977, p. 281.
4. W. E. Connor and S. L. Connor, *Prev. Med.*, **1**, 49 (1972).
5. C. B. Taylor, D. E. Patton, G. E. Cox, *Arch. Path.*, **76**, 404 (1963).
6. M. L. Armstrong, E. D. Warner, W. E. Connor, *Circ. Res.*, **27**, 59 (1961).
7. W. E. Connor, R. E. Hodges, and R. E. Bleiler, *J. Lab. Clin. Med.*, **57**, 331 (1961).
8. W. E. Connor, R. E. Hodges, and R. E. Bleiler, *J. Clin Invest.*, **40**, 894 (1961).
9. W. E. Connor, D. B. Stone, and R. E. Hodges, *J. Clin. Invest.*, **43**, 1691 (1964).
10. J. M. R. Beveridge, W. F. Connell, G. A. Mayer, et al., *J. Nutr.*, **71**, 61 (1960).
11. A. Steiner, E. J. Howard, and S. Akgun, *J.A.M.A.*, **181**, 186 (1962).
12. W. E. Connor and D. S. Lin, *J. Clin. Invest.*, **53**, 1062 (1974).
13. A. K. Bhattacharyya, W. E. Connor, F. A. Mausolf, et al., *J. Lab. Clin Med.*, **87**, 503 (1976).
14. W. E. Connor and S. N. Jagannathan, *Ann. Int. Med.*, abstract, **78**, 820 (1973).
15. R. W. Mahley, *Disturbances in Lipid and Lipoprotein Metabolism*, The American Physiological Society, 181 (1978).
16. W. E. Connor, *Proceedings of the Second Int. Symposium on Atherosclerosis*, 253, (1970).
17. E. H. Ahrens, J. Hirsch, and W. Insull, *Lancet*, **1**, 943 (1957).
18. A. Keys, J. T. Anderson, and F. Grande, *Lancet*, **1**, 787 (1957).
19. D. B. Zilversmit, *Cir. Res.*, **33**, 633 (1973).
20. D. M. Hegsted, R. B. McGandy, M. L. Myers, and F. J. Stare, *Am. J. Clin. Nutr.*, **17**, 281 (1965).
21. A. Keys, J. T. Anderson, and F. Grande, *Lancet*, **2**, 959 (1957).
22. W. E. Connor, D. T. Witiak, D. B. Stone, et al., *J. Clin. Invest.*, **48**, 1363 (1969).
23. R. A. J. Sturdevant, M. L. Pearce, and S. Dayton, *N. Engl. J. Med.*, **288**, 24 (1973).
24. F. Ederer, P. Lerent, O. Turpeninen, et al., *Lancet*, **2**, 203 (1971).
25. J. Olefsky, G. M. Reaven, and J. W. Farquhar, *J. Clin. Invest.*, **53**, 64 (1974).
26. W. B. Galbraith, W. E. Connor, D. B. Stone, *Ann. Intern. Med.*, **64**, 268 (1966).

27. E. H. Ahrens, J. Hirsch, K. Ottle, et al., *Trans. Assoc. Am. Phys.*, **74,** 134 (1961). (1961).

28. W. E. Connor, A. A. Spector, D. B. Stone, et al., *Circ. (Supple. III),* **40,** 61 (1969).

29. W. E. Connor, M. M. Fry, S. L. Connor, Unpublished data.

30. A. Antonis and I. Behrson, *Lancet,* **1,** 3 (1961).

31. D. B. Stone and W. E. Connor, *Diabetes,* **12,** 127 (1963).

32. R. L. Weinsier, A. Seeman, M. G. Herrera, et al., *Ann. Int. Med.,* **80,** 332 (1974).

33. W. E. Connor and M. M. Fry, Unpublished data.

34. P. J. Barter, K. F. Carroll, and P. J. Nestel, *J. Clin. Invest.,* **50,** 583 (1971).

35. J. Yudkin and L. Roddy, *Lancet,* **2,** 6 (1964).

36. I. MacDonald and D. W. Braithwaite, *Clin. Sci.,* **27,** 23 (1964).

37. T. F. Dunnigan, M. T. McKiddie, and S. M. Crosbie, *Clin. Sci.,* **38,** 1 (1970).

38. A. Keys, J. T. Anderson, and F. Grande, *J. Nutr.,* **70,** 257 (1960).

39. J. A. Little, B. L. Birchwood, D. A. Simmons, et al., *Atherosclerosis,* **II,** 173 (1970).

40. F. Grande, J. T. Anderson, and A. Keys, *J. Nutr.,* **86,** 313 (1965).

41. A. Keys, F. Grande, and J. T. Anderson, *Proc. Soc. Exp. Biol.,* **106,** 555 (1961).

42. T. L. Raymond, W. E. Connor, D. S. Lin, S. Warner, M. M. Fry, and S. L. Connor, *J. Clin. Invest.,* **60,** 1429 (1977).

43. D. P. Burkitt, A. R. P. Walker, and N. S. Painter, *J.A.M.A.,* **229,** 1068 (1974).

44. M. T. Cerqueira, M. McMurry-Fry, and W. E. Connor, *Am. J. Clin. Nutr.* (in press, 1978).

45. H. Trowell, *Am. J. Clin. Nutr.,* **25,** 926 (1972).

46. C. S. Leiber, D. P. Jones, J. Mendelson, et al., *Trans. Assoc. Am. Physicians,* **76,** 289 (1967).

47. D. J. Kudzma and G. Schonfeld, *J. Lab Clin. Med.,* **77,** 384 (1971).

48. M. S. Losowsky, D. P. Jones, C. S. Davidson, et al., *Am. J. Med.,* **35,** 794 (1963).

49. H. Ginsberg, J. Olefsky, J. W. Farquhar, et al., *Ann. Intern. Med.,* **80,** 143 (1974).

50. W. E. Connor, S. L. Connor, M. M. Fry-McMurry, and S. Warner, *The Alternative Diet Book,* Univ. Of Iowa Press, Iowa City, Iowa, 1976.

51. M. J. Mellies. T. T. Ishikawa, C. J. Glueck, et al., *J. Lab. Clin. Med.,* **88,** 914, (1976).

Lipids in Cystic Fibrosis

13

Lipids in Cystic Fibrosis

MARY LORETTA ROSENLUND and
EDWARD P. WALSH

Children's Hospital of Philadelphia, Pennsylvania

and

DANIEL A. SCOTT and DAVID KRITCHEVSKY

Wistar Institute of Anatomy and Biology, Philadelphia, Pennsylvania

Cystic fibrosis (CF) is one of the most common genetic diseases of the Caucasian race, occurring in about one of every 1600 live births. It is believed to be an autosomal recessive disease with one of every twenty people carrying the gene. The principal manifestations of CF are intestinal malabsorption, frequent and often severe respiratory infections, impaired growth, impaired reproduction, and a characteristic defect in sweat reabsorption that results in an excessive amount of sodium and chloride in sweat. As yet there is no known cause of CF, and no cure. It is not possible to identify a carrier until a child is born with CF; its parents are then recognized as obligate heterozygotes for the disease. A recent review indicates that the incidence of CF is becoming more frequent, with the number of adults receiving care at CF centers increasing at the rate of 200 patients per year (1).

In the approximately forty years since CF was first recognized as a disease entity we have learned much about its treatment, including supplementation of the diet with pancreatic enzymes, multivitamins, and additional salt, and the use of chest physiotherapy and antibiotics. It has become possible to add years to the average life span of CF patients, but

Supported in part by grants RR-00240(CRI) and AG-00076 and Research Career Award HL-0734 from the National Institutes of Health; from the Cystic Fibrosis Foundation, and from Best Foods, a division of CPC International, Inc.

we have not yet reached an equilibrium between the disease and the environment.

There are certain aspects of the symptomatology of CF that bear a resemblance to those of essential fatty acid (EFA) deficiency (Table 1). In 1929 Burr and Burr demonstrated that linoleic acid was an essential dietary component (2). Diets deficient in this EFA resulted in growth failure, elevated metabolic rate, increased caloric consumption, extreme emaciation, scaly skin, and impairment of reproductive capacity in rats. An increase in permeability of skin capillaries has also been observed in rats (3). Puppies fed a low fat diet were especially susceptible to respiratory infections (4). Human infants fed diets low in EFA suffered many of the same effects, as well as diarrhea (5). All symptoms, in animals and humans, were correctable when the subject received a diet containing sufficient EFAs.

Elliot and his colleagues (6,7) found that intravenous administration of EFA seemed to affect certain aspects of the CF. However, their sample was small and data were limited. We elected to feed a group of patients essential fatty acids orally since intravenous administration is not a practical method for long term treatment.

Our initial study involved 13 patients for a 1-year period, and these had varying degrees of CF, as determined by the Shwachman rating (8). This method of assessing the severity of the disease is based on four parameters: general activity, physical examination, nutritional status, and chest X-ray, each valued at 25 points. The higher the score, the better the prognosis. This scoring system allows a generalized assessment, and is helpful in determining the course of a patient's disease over long periods of time. If a patient goes to school regularly and has full normal activity, he or she gets 25 points for general ability; if he or she falls below the third percentile in height and weight and has bulky, fatty stools, the score for nutrition is only 10, and so forth.

Table 1   Similarities between Cystic Fibrosis and Essential Fatty Acid Deficiency

Symptom	CF	EFA Deficiency
Failure to thrive	+	+
Increased metabolic rate	+	+
Diarrhea/steatorrhea	+	+
Respiratory infections	+	+
Impaired reproductive capacity	+	+

**Table 2   Patients Participating in
1-Year Corn Oil Feeding Trial**

Patient	Sex	Age (years)	Shwachman Rating
LB	F	6½	50
ME	M	9½	80
KF	F	5	60
MG	F	3	65
SL	M	11	80
WL	F	13½	75
ML	M	10½	55
JL	M	2½	90
CL	F	3	60
DP	F	10	90
RR	F	11½	85
MS	F	5½	85
EV	M	4	70

Because patients with CF have varying degrees of involvement, the patients were their own controls, with all parameters from the year prior to the study evaluated against the study year. Table 2 lists the patients, their ages at the start of the study, sex, and state of disease as determined by the Shwachman rating. Although none of the children was severely ill, two children had moderately severe disease, four had mild disease, five were rated as good, and two as excellent.

Baseline data were obtained prior to the dietary trial. After the initial studies, all of the patients received EFA orally in the form of corn oil (1 gm/kg/day). This was given with meals, along with vitamin E (10 mg/kg/day with no dose greater than 200 mg/day) four times a day, for 1 year. Since we were adding large levels of polyunsaturated fatty acids to the diet, we added vitamin E for its antioxidant properties.

Records were kept of height and weight, number of respiratory infections, as well as antibiotic courses, number and type of stools, and number of pancreatic enzyme capsules required per day. During this year, the patients continued their regular treatment program, which consisted of pulmonary physiotherapy at least twice a day, multivitamins, dietary pancreatic enzymes and salt supplementation, plus the use of antibiotics as indicated. Other than the addition of EFA and vitamin E to the diet, there was no change in treatment from the year prior to the study in any of the children. They continued to be seen by the same physicians in the Cystic Fibrosis Clinic at Children's Hospital of Philadelphia.

Results of the study were varied. Although some response was noted in all patients, there were no consistent clinical changes seen in every patient. The amount of pancreatic enzyme supplements had to be increased initially with EFA treatment for all but one patient. However, the stools decreased in number or remained the same in 11 patients. Stool trypsin, after 1 year of EFA treatment, reverted to normal in three patients. All but two patients gained weight during the study year, but the increase was not significant. Every patient gained in height, three moving to higher percentiles. The average Shwachman rating was unchanged, however (Table 3).

The oral EFA therapy effected no change in sputum cultures, although five families felt the patients had fewer respiratory infections. White blood counts returned to or towards normal in nine of the 13 patients. Chest X-rays showed no significant changes, and pulmonary function studies showed decline in some patients and improvement in others. Most important, there was no clinical deterioration noted in any of the 13 patients during the time of oral EFA administration.

One consistent change in all patients was the sweat sodium concentration, as seen in Table 3. Levels prior to oral EFA administration were all above 100 meq/L, diagnostic of CF. After one year of EFA, the sweat sodium concentration was lower in all but one patient (ML) whose sodium remained the same. The average decrease was significant at the 1% level. The sweat sodium determinations were carried out on samples of at least 100 mg of sweat using the Gibson-Cook method of collection. There were two patients with exceptionally high sweat sodium levels (CL and SL). In their cases, we collected 278 and

Table 3 Influence of Corn Oil Feeding on Shwachman Rating, Sweat Sodium (meq/L), Serum T3 and T4 in CF Patients (Average ± SEM of 13 patients)

	Before Treatment	After Treatment
Shwachman rating	72.7 ± 3.8	73.6 ± 3.8
Sweat sodium	147.5 ± 13.0	99.6 ± 6.9[a]
T3	68.6 ± 3.6	50.3 ± 2.2[b]
T4	9.3 ± 0.6	9.3 ± 0.9

[a] $p < 0.01$.
[b] $p < 0.001$.

192 mg of sweat, respectively. The change in sweat sodium concentration, excluding these patients, was still significant, but none of the levels fell within the normal range.

Because of the increased metabolism and poor growth often seen in CF, we studied thyroid function in these children (Table 3). Levels of T4 were normal in all patients at the outset and did not change. However, T3 was elevated above a normal level in seven of the subjects prior to EFA treatment, and was within normal range in all subjects after 1 year of oral administration of EFA. This may be related to the increased serum proteins found in all patients after EFA treatment. Serum albumin levels did not change as a result of treatment, but serum globulin levels were significantly elevated (2.63 ± 0.24 versus 3.75± 0.17) ($p < 0.001$).

After the recent report that EFAs were absorbed through the skin, we had one mother rub a tablespoon of corn oil into the skin of her CF baby, whose serum EFAs were low, four times a day. Three months later, his serum EFA spectrum was normal, he had gained significantly in height and weight, and was no longer having respiratory difficulty.

The clinical aspect of our study is small, but promising. The results suggest a role for EFAs in the care of CF. Whether EFA is a factor in the etiology of CF or merely a manifestation of malabsorption requires further investigation.

There have been a number of investigations into the nature of the serum lipids in CF. Kuo and Huang (10) found that serum cholesterol and phospholipid levels were significantly lower in CF patients but that triglyceride levels were similar in CF patients and controls. Analysis of the fatty acid spectra of serum triglycerides, cholesteryl ester, lecithin, and free fatty acids showed that linoleic acid was significantly higher in all fractions of normal serum, and arachidonic acid was higher in cholesteryl esters of normal serum. Palmitic, palmitoleic, and oleic acids predominated in CF serum. Caren and Corbo (11) compared sera of 23 CF patients with those of 8 controls with results similar to those of Kuo and Huang. Wiese and co-workers (12) also found that serum cholesterol levels of CF patients were significantly lower than those of controls. They found that CF serum had significantly higher levels of saturated and monoenoic fatty acids and significantly lower levels of linoleic acid but found no differences in arachidonic acid content of normal or CF sera. Underwood, Denning, and Navab (13) found a similar pattern in CF sera except that their patients had higher serum arachidonic acid levels than the controls. Bennett and Medwadowski (14) confirmed the observation of Wiese et al. (12) and also found that CF sera contained lower levels of vitamins A and E. Our own initial analysis of the serum

Table 4   Influence of Corn Oil Feeding on Serum Fatty Acid Spectra in 13 CF Patients (Values represent % change from starting levels after 1 year of treatment)[a]

	Serum Fraction		
Fatty Acid	Cholesteryl Ester	Triglyceride	Phospholipid
Lauric (12:0)	−23	+21	—
Palmitic (16:0)	−33	+8	+5
Palmitoleic (16:1)	−16	−26	—
Stearic (18:0)	−100	−60	−24
Oleic (18:1)	−25	NC	−40
Linoleic (18:2)	+92	+54	+106
Arachidonic (20:4)	+95	NC	+96

[a] NC = no change.

fatty acids of CF patients (15) was in accord with the earlier work. To date there have been no reports of the effects of CF on distribution and composition of serum lipoproteins. Such studies, when available, may shed more light on the nature of lipid transport in CF.

The influence of corn oil feeding upon the serum fatty acid spectra of our CF patients is presented in Table 4. The significant effect of this regimen on serum linoleic and arachidonic acid levels is evident. The clinical effects of this regimen (16) were discussed earlier in this presentation.

We have now followed a number of corn oil-treated CF patients for more than 2 years and the alterations in their serum fatty acid patterns have been maintained. The effect of this regimen on the cholesteryl ester fatty acids is shown in Table 5.

In every analysis of individual fatty acids of CF sera the significant increase in palmitoleic acid content is evident (10,11,15).

Administration of corn oil to CF patients tends to normalize serum palmitoleic acid levels (Table 6). The role of palmitoleic acid in the progression of CF or possibly in its early detection becomes important. Palmitoleic acid accumulates in livers of rats rendered EFA-deficient (17,18). Although palmitoleic acid could theoretically be elongated and further desaturated to give a 20-carbon atom, tetraunsaturated isomer of arachidonic acid, very little of this polyunsaturated fatty acid actually accumulates (19). One reason for the lack of build-up of the tetraenoic acid (4,7,10,13–20:4) is the very slow desaturation of palmitoleic acid

Table 5   Influence of Corn Oil Therapy on Fatty Acids of Serum Cholesteryl Esters (Patients on therapy 1½–2 years)

Group	No.	Fatty Acid (%) ± SEM[a]		
		18:1	18:2	20:4
Control	15	23.2 ± 1.0a	47.5 ± 2.7c	5.3 ± 0.7
CF (untreated)	15	30.1 ± 2.7ab	32.7 ± 3.6c	3.2 ± 1.6
CF (treated)	14	21.9 ± 0.8b	40.5 ± 2.7	5.1 ± 0.9

[a] Values bearing same letter are significantly different.

to the corresponding C16 dienoic acid. Palmitoleic can also be converted to vaccenic acid (18:1 ω 11) but no attempts have been made to identify this acid in CF serum.

A possible approach to delineation of the role of palmitoleic acid in CF is to examine its occurrence and metabolism in CF skin fibroblasts in tissue culture.

Drs. George H. Rothblat and Marguerita de la Llera of the Medical College of Pennsylvania in Philadelphia have successfully maintained a strain of fibroblast cells developed from a skin biopsy taken from a CF patient. When these cells were grown in a medium containing delipidized serum protein, their fatty acid spectrum was significantly different from that of cells grown in 20% fetal calf serum (Table 7). Cells grown in delipidized serum protein contained significantly more palmitoleic acid, less arachidonic, and no linoleic. The fatty acids of the cells grown in fetal calf serum were undoubtedly derived from that serum (20). Whether normal cells grown under lipid-free conditions give rise to a

Table 6   Influence of Corn Oil Therapy (1½–2 years) on Palmitoleic Acid Content of Serum Total Fatty Acids in CF Patients

Group	No.	Palmitoleic Acid (%) ± SEM[a]
Control	15	1.01 ± 0.35a
CF (untreated)	15	5.44 ± 0.63ab
CF (treated)	14	0.97 ± 0.27b

[a] Values bearing same letter are significantly different.

Table 7   Fatty Acid Spectra of CF Fibroblasts Grown in Culture Medium Containing Fetal Calf Serum (FCS) on Delipidized Serum Protein (DLP)

	Percent ± SEM	
Fatty Acid	DLP 8 Samples: Passage 6–10	FCS 4 Samples: Passage 8–10
Lauric (12:0)	0.28 ± 0.02	0.32 ± 0.02
Myristic (14:0)	3.50 ± 0.09	2.77 ± 0.05[a]
Palmitic (16:0)	24.88 ± 0.53	26.53 ± 0.44[a]
Palmitoleic (16:1)	4.34 ± 0.23	0.48 ± 0.48[b]
Stearic (18:0)	52.60 ± 1.53	56.90 ± 1.00[a]
Oleic (18:1)	12.77 ± 1.57	8.60 ± 1.36
Linoleic (18:2)	0	0.84 ± 0.26[b]
Arachidonic (20:4)	1.63 ± 0.44	3.57 ± 0.28[c]

[a] $p < 0.05$.
[b] $p < 0.001$.
[c] $p < 0.01$.

fatty acid spectrum similar to that seen in the CF fibroblasts awaits results from experiments that are currently under way.

REFERENCES

1. W. J. Warwick and R. E. Pogue, *J.A.M.A.*, **238,** 2159 (1977).
2. G. O. Burr and M. M. Burr, *J. Biol. Chem.*, **86,** 587 (1930).
3. J. Kramar and V. E. Levine, *J. Nutrition*, **50,** 149 (1953).
4. A. E. Hansen and H. F. Wiese, *Texas Rep. Biol. Med.*, **9,** 491 (1951).
5. A. E. Hansen, *Pediatrics*, **21,** 171 (1963).
6. R. B. Elliott, *Pediatric Res.*, **7,** 427 (1973).
7. R. B. Elliott, *Pediatrics*, **57,** 474 (1976).
8. H. Shwachman and L. L. Kulczycki, *Am. J. Dis. Child.*, **96,** 6 (1958).
9. L. E. Gibson and R. E. Cooke, *Pediatrics*, **23,** 545 (1959).
10. P. T. Kuo and N. N. Huang, *J. Clin. Invest.*, **44,** 1924 (1965).
11. R. Caren and L. Corbo, *J. Clin. Endocrinol. Metab.*, **26,** 470 (1966).
12. H. F. Wiese, M. J. Bennett, I. H. G. Braun, W. Yamanaka, and E. Coon, *Am. J. Clin. Nutr.*, **18,** 155 (1966).

13. B. A. Underwood, C. R. Denning, and M. Navab, *Ann. N.Y. Acad. Sci.,* **203,** 237 (1972).

14. M. J. Bennett and B. F. Medwadowski, *Am. J. Clin. Nutr.,* **20,** 415 (1967).

15. M. L. Rosenlund, H. K. Kim, and D. Kritchevsky, *Nature* **251,** 719 (1974).

16. M. L. Rosenlund, J. A. Selekman, H. K. Kim, and D. Kritchevsky, *Pediatrics,* **59,** 428 (1977).

17. H. Mohrhauer and R. T. Holman, *J. Lipid Res.,* **4,** 151 (1963).

18. R. O. Peluffo, A. M. Nervi, and R. R. Brenner, *Biochim. Biophys. Acta.,* **441,** 25 (1976).

19. H. Sprecher, in *Polyunsaturated Fatty Acids,* W. H. Kunau and R. T. Holman, Eds., Am. Oil Chem. Soc., Champaign, Ill., 1977, pp. 1–18.

20. B. V. Howard and D. Kritchevsky, *Biochim. Biophys. Acta,* **187,** 293 (1969).

Index